HERBAL HEALING
for children

A PARENT'S GUIDE TO TREATMENTS FOR COMMON CHILDHOOD ILLNESSES

Demetria Clark

Healthy Living Publications
Summertown Tennessee

Library of Congress Cataloging-in-Publication Data

Clark, Demetria.
   Herbal healing for children : a parent's guide to treatments for common
childhood illnesses / Demetria Clark.
      p. cm.
   Includes bibliographical references and index.
   ISBN 978-1-57067-214-9
   1. Herbs—Therapeutic use—Popular works.   2. Children—Diseases—
Alternative treatment—Popular works.   I. Title.
   RJ53.H47C53 2010
   615'.3210835—dc22   2010042693

Book Publishing Company is a member of Green Press Initiative. We chose to print this
title on paper with 100% postconsumer recycled content, processed without chlorine,
which saves the following natural resources:

BOOK
PUBLISHING
COMPANY

green
press
INITIATIVE

- 33 trees
- 917 pounds of solid waste
- 15, 105 gallons of water
- 3,136 pounds of greenhouse gases
- 10 million BTU of energy

For more information on Green Press Initiative, visit www.greenpressinitiative.org.

Environmental impact estimates were made using the Environmental Defense Fund Paper
Calculator. For more information visit www.papercalculator.org.

Printed on recycled paper

This book is not to be used as a replacement for medical guidance. It is not intended as
medi-cal advice. Using herbal remedies may involve some risk. Because of this, the author,
writer, publisher, and/or distributors of this book are not responsible for any adverse
effects resulting from the use of the herbal remedies described herein. If your child has
been diagnosed with any illness or condition, consult with your doctor or health-care
practitioner before using herbal remedies.
   Review the information and assess all information and formulations for use for
your family. Do not use a remedy or an herb if you suspect or believe it will not be the
proper application.

Published by Healthy Living Publications,
an imprint of Book Publishing Company
P.O. Box 99
Summertown, TN 38483
888-260-8458 • www.bookpubco.com

ISBN 978-1-57067-214-9

Printed in Canada

17 16 15 14 13 12 11   9 8 7 6 5 4 3 2 1

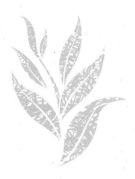

To all the families with questions
and the parents who want to find another way,
and to all the people who believe
that nature nurtures.

contents

foreword

ike the nurturing mother she is, Demetria has gathered her herbal wisdom and her many years of experience as a parent and community herbalist and set it forth in this imminently practical and useful book on herbal caregiving for children. She calls it a "gentle guidebook"—and it *is* gentle, safe, and easy to follow— but it's also richly enlivened with Demetria's passion and love for the plants. As she shares in the opening line of the introduction, "I did not come to herbalism; herbalism came to me." As a young child growing up in the bush of Alaska, she knew clearly what she wanted to be and do with her life, something truly rare in our day and age when even adults often don't discover their true passion in life until they are much older. Plants and healing herbs claimed Demetria from an early age, and they became a way of life for her. Her lifetime experience using herbs for daily health and healing both as a community practitioner and a family herbalist shines through in the pages of this book.

There are endless good recipes, tips on keeping our children healthy, instructions on how to make your own herbal remedies, an overview of the historical and traditional basis of herbal medicine, along with an in-depth discussion of the safety issues of using herbal remedies for children. But what makes Dementria's book so special and readable is the rich interweaving of her personal stories and experiences both as a parent and as a practicing herbalist.

Reading *Herbal Healing for Children* is like sitting down with a wise, old herbalist over a cup of steaming tea and having a personal consult or friendly chat. "What do I do for my child's ear infection or a high persistent fever?" you might ask. Demetria offers not only an explanation of what might be the underlying cause of the imbalance, but also lists several effective herbal remedies that are known to work well. Most of the remedies are simple, cost effective, and easily doable. Some are found in the kitchen cupboard or growing in your garden. And like any wise healer, always thinking of the child first, she offers cautions and guidelines for when it might be necessary to call in a doctor or other health-care professional. When unsure of what to do, Demetria kindly directs us where to find an answer either through an extensive resource list or through the plants' own gentle guidance.

Like the earth goddess for whom she's named, Demetria fills us with her earthly wisdom and practical advice: "Herbs are a gift from the earth. Just as parents are natural healers, herbs are natural medicines." and "Humans are not mere tenders of the natural world but are an integral part of it, and the natural world is an integral part of us." So grab a cup of tea, pick up this trusty book, and enjoy. What you'll readily find is a safe, gentle introduction to the use of herbs for children and the sacred tradition of herbalism.

Rosemary Gladstar
herbalist and author of *Herbal Healing for Women*

acknowledgments

Thank you to all of my students, who taught me more than I could ever imagine, and who accepted me for my passion and in spite of my shortcomings. I have been blessed to be involved with all of you.

I am grateful to my lifelong friends and family: Annie, thank you for understanding and being my dear, wonderful friend. John, you are a source of intellectual sparring, old-time life memories, and friendship—thank you for keeping the link. Wendy, thank you for sharing memories and for being an incredible friend, mother, and woman. Kathy, you are wild, wise, and lovely, and a perpetual beacon. Angel, thank you for singing, for being no man's rib, and for being a person of trust in a strange world. Carol, thank you for being a friend and for sharing the spirit of innovation with me. Barry, thank you for being you, saying it straight, and being an incredible father-in-law. Kathy, I appreciate you so much. Joe, thank you for teaching me to work for what I know is right and to follow through on my passion. Mom, thank you for teaching me about passion and for sharing with me your belief that love will change the world. Gretchen, I am grateful that you are my opposite and that you help me to see the other side of things. Griffin, thank you for being a strong man and a good father. Lanny, you combine the best of wit and wisdom and give me hope for the future. Michael, you are an inspiration and a beacon of hope. Grampa, you are a true friend and a man about whom books should be written. Gramma, you are the original power woman: hip, smart, talented, and compassionate to all. Andrew, you speak to my soul, sing my soul song, and make me know happiness. Jacob and Taro, no mother could be prouder, happier, or more in love with her children.

I am grateful to my many teachers: Rosemary Gladstar, know that I always cherish your works and words in the very depths of my soul. Susun Weed, thank you for offering exactly what I needed when I needed it; your encouragement means so much. Ina May Gaskin, thank you for being a friend and teacher from whom I have gleaned so much knowledge. I also extend a special acknowledgment to all of my other teachers at The Farm: Pamela, Deborah, Carol, and Sharon. Thank you all!

Carol Wiley Lorente, editor extraordinaire, thank you. I feel so strongly that this partnership was meant to be. You assisted me in formatting my rambling thoughts and ideas, and came up with an excellent manuscript. From the start, you believed in this work and believed in me. Thank you from the bottom of my heart.

Introduction

I did not come to herbalism; herbalism came to me. The natural world has always fascinated me. When I was a child, my family moved often. I spent my childhood playing in diverse landscapes in Alabama, Alaska, New Hampshire, North Carolina, and Oregon. Every time we settled in a new area, I would be struck by the stark differences in the plants and trees. Running through fields, rolling in the grass and weeds, making the usual childhood crowns and bracelets from plants, and disappearing into herbs and flowers taller than I was were powerful introductions to the natural world that always surrounded me.

Living in Alaska probably did more to clinch my choice of a future occupation than anything else. Several things happened to me there that cemented my interest in herbs and put me on my life's path.

I had assumed Alaska was all snow and igloos, but we moved to wild and beautiful Kodiak Island, most of which is a nature preserve. It wasn't just the herbs and plants growing there that left an impression on me. We were a military family living among other military families, so my childhood chums represented a diverse mix of ethnic groups. I started to observe what families did to stay healthy. The herbal traditions of Africans, Inuit, Puerto Ricans, and others became part of my frame of reference and way of life.

When I was eight, my mother got a job in a health-food store, and I became a vegetarian. I began to read about food, herbs, and plants. Even as a young girl, I was attracted to old pharmacopeias. The beauty of herbs drew me into the study of herbal medicine. While other children talked about what they wanted to be when they grew up, I never really felt that I had a choice other than herbalism.

Throughout my childhood, I was regularly exposed to the healing power of plants and herbs. Friends in Alabama explained that collard greens are high in iron, so they ate them often because their child was anemic. Our neighbors in New Hampshire owned an herbal-therapy company. This wonderful family offered me real guidance and answered all of what I am sure were my annoying and endless questions about herbs. I remember badgering my friend's mom about why she grew certain herbs and used certain essential oils. I also remember going to their essential oils warehouse for the first time and feeling like I had reached olfactory heaven. Smelling all of the herbs and essential oils was an amazing experience that I've never forgotten. (I still purchase herbs and oils from them.)

All of these experiences impressed me. But a personal experience with chronic migraines totally convinced me of the effectiveness of herbs. As a child, I had such severe migraines that I'd have nosebleeds. The pain felt like a hammer smacking into my head, and the bleeding was, of course, frightening. Yet no doctor seemed to be able to help me. I remember, at the tender age of eight, using cool compresses, taking baths, and swallowing three, four, or even five aspirins at a time in a vain attempt to quell the pain. Then I had what I call my "herbal encounter."

One day, my head pounding from a migraine, I ran to the stream near our house and dunked my head in the cold water to cool off. I then walked in the woods along the stream, even though I was feeling very sick. Without knowing why, I absentmindedly began chewing on a leaf of mountain laurel that I'd picked along the stream and, to my surprise, I began to feel better. I learned later, as an adult, that mountain laurel was an old headache remedy that can be highly toxic if not used properly. But as a child, I naively believed that plants, being "natural," could not hurt me. Mountain laurel became part of my personal materia medica, and I learned how to stop the headaches and nosebleeds. Learning how herbs worked helped me understand why I had migraines and how I could change the outcome.

All of this exposure and my love of plants started to click. Herbs and plants as medicine became my lifelong love and interest. I began my formal herbalism training at age thirteen. Over the years, I have been lucky enough to have studied with renowned herbalists, such as Rosemary Gladstar, Christopher Hobbs, David Hoffmann, Jane

Smolnik, Susun Weed, David Winston, and scores of other amazing teachers. I have taken many graduate-level courses in botany, forestry, horticulture, and nutrition. I was on the faculty of the Midwives College of Utah. And I have studied aromatherapy at the Pacific Institute of Aromatherapy and with Jeanne Rose.

I went on the road with the Grateful Dead as a Deadhead, making herbal teas, aromatherapy lotions, and remedies for those traveling with us and for anyone else who needed help. We didn't always have access to health care, so this knowledge was beneficial to me and my friends as we dealt with issues such as burns, morning sickness, muscle aches, premenstrual syndrome (PMS), and stomach bugs. (Although I have met members of the band and once made a remedy basket as a gift for Bob Weir, I was not their herbalist—I don't know how that rumor got started!)

In 1998, I founded my herbal training school, Heart of Herbs, and have since trained thousands of students in the art of herbal medicine. (One of my students had enlisted my services years ago while we were all on the road with the Dead).

When I had children, it seemed natural to use herbs to treat their various illnesses. Lately, more and more parents are coming to me for counseling. They are frightened and disenchanted with the harsh medications given to their children for common illnesses. Are there alternatives, they ask, to high-powered antibiotics? Now that many children's cold medicines have been deemed dangerous or, at the very least, useless, what can we do to make our children comfortable while they recover from the common cold? What can we give our child for a tummy ache? Do we really need an expensive prescription antifungal cream for our baby's diaper rash?

At a time when an increasing number of families lack health insurance or adequate coverage, more and more parents are turning to herbal medicines to treat their children. Parents know many common childhood illnesses and conditions do not necessarily require the inevitable long waits in doctors' offices or prescriptions for powerful, expensive medicines. They want something gentler that won't break the bank but will still help their children feel better and get well.

Many parents are raising their children with a more holistic lifestyle. These families often eat organic foods and grow their own vegetables. They are environmentally conscious. And they are looking for safer, simpler, and more natural ways to care for their children.

What could be a better choice than using herbal remedies to treat their children's illnesses?

Children seem to thrive and have fewer side effects when they are given herbs rather than conventional medications. I have seen children show marked improvement after only one or two doses of an herbal remedy, even after there had been no improvement with standard medicines. I once treated a child who had repeated bouts of bronchitis, and obtained good results after modifying the child's diet (eliminating meat and dairy products) and administering five doses of an effective herbal tea that contained both medicinal and nutritional properties.

The purpose of this book is to empower parents, to give them safe and effective alternatives to potent medicines whose side effects can often make their children feel worse, and to help parents take control of their children's recovery from illness. Parents know their children better than anyone. They have what I call a primal inkling: they know how their children behave when they aren't feeling well, and they know their children's energy levels, eating habits, and sleeping habits. When you use this book, I encourage you to reconnect with that parental instinct but, of course, don't forget to employ common sense.

This book is an easy-to-follow, hands-on, practical guide to alternative medications for common childhood health issues: easy teas for a tummy ache, drops for earaches, treatments for eczema and diaper rash, and much more. This is a gentle guidebook, not a promotion of any sort of dogma. If you have chosen this book, you are already interested in alternatives, and I want you to have a safe, informative place to find what you need.

After an introduction to herbal medicine in chapter 1, I discuss commonly used herbs in chapter 2 and explain why each herb works and what conditions it is prescribed for. Chapter 2 also lists important information about herbs that you should always have on hand and those that can be dangerous for children.

Chapter 3 is the guts of the book, where you will turn for guidance when your little one is under the weather or awakens with a feverish cry in the middle of the night. Illnesses are listed in alphabetical order, with remedies immediately following. Remedies for the illnesses call for herbs and herbal products that can be purchased in natural-food stores, online, or from the companies listed under Suppliers, pages 191–194.

Ready-made and readily available herbs and herb products make it easy and simple to administer herbal medicines at home. But if you'd like to make your own remedies, chapter 4 will tell you how and where to buy or gather herbs, and how to preserve and store them. Chapter 5 will teach you how to make your own decoctions, herbal teas, infusions, and salves. Chapter 6 includes recipes for some of my favorite and most popular remedies, which can be made and kept on hand so they're always available when you need them.

At the back of the book, you will find additional information, such as where to buy herbs, how to grow your own (including several herb garden designs), where to find an herbalist, and which books to keep in your library.

Herbs are a gift from the earth. Just as parents are natural healers, herbs are natural medicines. In a time when parents know more names of prescription drugs than of plants, we need natural remedies for our children more than ever.

An Introduction to Herbalism

T he world of herbal medicine is a vast network of practitioners, botanists, historians, teachers, and researchers whose compendium of knowledge guides most of the world's population in curing illness and staying healthy. The World Health Organization recently estimated that more than 80 percent of the world's population relies on herbal medicines for some portion of it's primary health care. In Germany and Switzerland, roughly six to seven hundred plant-based medicines are available and are prescribed by approximately 70 percent of physicians. In many parts of Europe, herbals are blended and compounded in the apothecary where prescription medicines are also sold.

During the past twenty years in the United States, the public has become increasingly dissatisfied with the cost, questionable safety, and lack of effectiveness of prescription medications. This dissatisfaction, combined with an interest in returning to natural remedies, has led to a phenomenal resurgence in the use of herbal medicines. A 2001 study found that nearly 70 percent of Americans have used at least one form of alternative therapy in their lifetimes. This includes parents who are looking for safe, natural, and effective treatments for their children's common childhood illnesses rather than resorting to harsh prescription drugs. Indeed, alternative therapies represent one of the fastest growing sectors of American health care.

Herbalism is readily available to all who choose to use it. Because herbs are considered "food" and "supplements" by the U.S. Food and Drug Administration (FDA), herbs and herbal products can be found virtually everywhere—at drugstores, natural-food stores, supermarkets, and even gas station convenience stores. This ease of availability, however, can backfire if parents don't know the quality and content of what they are buying or don't know how to administer it to their children.

As a parent, you are in charge of your child's health. I use herbs exclusively in the treatment of my children's ills, and I have never been faced with a situation in which herbs have not worked for us. It is your right as a parent to decide how your child will be treated medically. I advise parents to educate themselves by reading, taking courses, or consulting an herbalist before they administer remedies. I also tell them to be sure to consult their physician or health-care practitioner before changing treatment.

Although this book is not a replacement for medical care, it can enlighten you about the option of treating common childhood illnesses with easily obtainable herbal products and remedies. It is designed to give you enough knowledge to talk confidently with your doctor or health-care practitioner and to help you take an active part in your child's health care.

WHY HERBS FOR KIDS?

We're facing a time when many once-trusted medications for children are now considered dangerous, when numerous drugs are being recalled or taken off the market, and when we are learning that some routinely prescribed medications have never actually been tested on children. It's no surprise, then, that parents are beginning to wonder where to turn. Herbal medicine offers parents another choice, particularly for treating common childhood illnesses, and it's an option that can be safe and effective, with thousands of years of knowledge behind it. Once you have researched herbal medicine and have a handle on which herbs do what, you'll be able to figure out which remedies to use simply by observing your child and paying attention to how he looks and behaves.

Treating a child with herbs can be an effective way to fortify the body and cure illness. Herbal medicine is the right choice for kids because it blends modern medical research with ancient practices and remedies. Children generally respond well to herbal remedies, even when they are administered in tiny doses. Children's bodies are sensitive and react promptly to an herb's synergistic, efficient, gentle effects.

An herbal remedy needs to be customized for each individual child. When I prescribe, I take into consideration the whole picture: the child's age and nutritional status, the family's lifestyle, and the home environment. It's like putting together a puzzle, with parents supplying the missing pieces.

A BRIEF HERBAL HISTORY

Unfortunately, most of us live in cultures that have forgotten the traditional practices and words of our elders. The realm of herbal healing, on the other hand, embraces ancient wisdom and cherishes the teachings, knowledge, and passions that our elders have transmitted to us.

For more than five thousand years, people have used various plant-based medicinal preparations to treat health disorders. These herbal pioneers recognized that humans are not mere tenders of the natural world but are an integral part of it, and the natural world is an integral part of us. Sadly, modern approaches have ignored the brilliance and practicality of early herbalists and have discounted their contributions to both herbal and traditional medicine.

Through a basic process of experimentation, these incredible pioneers began to collect and record their knowledge and remedies. They then handed them down to the next generation, noting which plants nourished a pregnant woman, for example, or soothed the nasty cough that seemed to hit their community every year in cold weather. The women and men who made medicine and healed their community members eventually became the medicine people, doctors, and master herbalists of their community or region.

Herbalism has not always been the practice we think of today. Rather, it was hands-on remedy making, based on healing practices not limited by definitions or governmental regulations. Its history is tightly intertwined with ancient medicine, modern medicine, and midwifery practices throughout the ages, and it has existed in almost all cultures of the world. Many of the first herbalists were women, mothers, and midwives. (As recently as just a hundred years ago, the woman of the house made most of her family's medicine, a tradition that is coming back into vogue as parents again take charge of their family's health.) Herbs were depicted with women in paintings and on coins, and they were even used as currency.

AN HERBAL TIMELINE

Herbal medicine was the people's medicine—it grew wherever they were. The practice of herbal medicine has been documented in ancient African, Chinese, Greek, Indian, Native American, Roman, and Tibetan cultures for thousands of years. Ultimately, the search for herbs led European explorers to seek and discover India and, by proxy, North America.

In Shanidar Cave in Iraq, pollen samples were found with human remains, indicating that Neanderthals who lived between 80,000–60,000 BP had been treated with herbal medicine. Remedies used at the time included bachelor's button, cornflower, grape hyacinth, hollyhock, yarrow, and other herbs.

Herbal medicine was used during the New Stone Age (8000–5000 BCE), when women gathered and men hunted. As the gatherers ventured forth for food each day, they took into account what was available and useful in their natural surroundings. Women practiced herbalism daily and were always on the lookout for what was growing and when it was at its peak of potency and nutrition.

The world's oldest surviving medical document, *Ebers Papyrus,* dates to 2000 BCE and lists medicinal prescriptions in use after about 1800 BCE. In the ancient libraries of the Achaemenid Dynasty (550–330 BCE), also known as the Persian Empire, there are texts containing lists of plants, herbs, and other substances used for medicinal purposes.

Although we know from recorded European history that herbal medicine was documented at the time of the Roman invasions, we also have anthropological evidence that herbs were used by the ancient Celts. Soutra Aisle, on the Scottish border, is believed to have been the site of one of the largest hospitals in the region during medieval times and dates from 1164 CE. Evidence of the use of hemlock, opium poppy, and other common herbs of the time has been unearthed there. An extremely important Welsh text, *The Red Book of Hergest* (circa 1425), described more than five hundred ways to use two hundred herbs. Herbs became such an important tool for healing that, in 1542, King Henry VIII signed a charter ensuring herbalists the right to practice.

During the battles of World War I, herbs were used for treating burns, preventing infections, and as antiseptics. In 1941, the government appealed to civilians to collect, grow, and identify herbs to be made into medicine. Today, British herbalists practice and are protected under the 1968 Medicines Act.

In the Americas, natives had used medicinal herbs for a thousand years before the Europeans arrived. They had accumulated a vast store of botanical and medical knowledge, a fact that surprised many European explorers. When the Europeans returned home, they took many native plants and Native American remedies. These became part of European herbal literature and practice.

Spiritual Healing

Throughout history, almost every culture has combined some aspect of spirituality, from a simple prayer to a shamanistic ritual, with healing. Healers have traditionally called upon the spiritual world to assist them in their work.

Today, many primitive tribes retain an expert knowledge of medicinal plants and their uses, and their plant "databases" can number into the hundreds. Contemporary herbalists have access to a great many texts by the elders of all nations. The world has a huge pharmacopoeia that is the basis for most of our modern pharmaceuticals.

USING HERBS SAFELY

Herbal remedies have stood the test of time. Herbalists are aware of which plants and remedies are tried and true, which ones to use for various purposes, and which ones to avoid. Yet parents invariably ask me whether herbal medicine is safe for babies and children. My answer is always the same: "Yes, but . . . ." As is the case for any medical treatment for your child, herbal medicine involves guidelines that must be followed, precautions that should be taken, and knowledge that should be gained before treatment begins.

Unfortunately, when we need to make decisions about our children's health, they are usually already in the throes of an illness. I tell parents that knowing about childhood illnesses before they hit, understanding their normal progression and healing patterns, and being knowledgeable about herbal medicines for kids will guide them in choosing safe and effective remedies when the moment arrives.

There's so much more involved in the issue of herbal safety than whether the herbs themselves are intrinsically harmless. Here is the advice I give to parents for using herbs safely:

Become familiar with primary childhood illnesses. These include chicken pox, colds, ear infections, fever, flu, tummy aches, and whooping cough (pertussis). In addition, get acquainted with the minor stuff, including bruises, bumps, cuts, sprains, and so on. Know what you're dealing with, so when you become familiar with herbs, you'll recognize which ones you'll need to use to treat the problem.

Learn about herbs and herbal medicine. Take classes, peruse websites, and read, read, read (see Recommended Reading, page 197). If you read only one or two books, I highly recommend *Herbal Therapy and Supplements: A Scientific and Traditional Approach* by Merrily A. Kuhn and David Winston and *Holistic Herbal* by David Hoffmann. Any other book that has a materia medica (a list of remedies and how they can be used) should be kept on hand so you can refer to it quickly.

Talk to your child's doctor or health-care practitioner. Discuss your intention to use herbal remedies, especially if your child is using prescription drugs. If the doctor does not know you are using herbal remedies, he may inadvertently prescribe a drug that interacts negatively with the herbs. In addition, if your child is taking prescription drugs, do not stop using the prescribed drugs and substitute herbal remedies without talking to your doctor.

Granted, it is your right as a parent to determine how your child should be treated medically, but it is essential that you foster an honest relationship with your child's doctor. I'm not saying you have to have the doctor's *approval* to use herbal remedies for your children, but he does need to know the whole story. An honest dialog can be an opportunity to educate your doctor. As a result of your discussion, he may become more open to herbal remedies and be more receptive when the next parents walk through the door. Better yet, your conversation may spark an interest in herbal medicine.

You may have to interview a few doctors before you find one who is supportive of herbal remedies for children. Many clients tell me they can't bring themselves to tell their doctors they're using herbal medicines because they are afraid of his reaction and of losing his support. Although I don't believe it's always intentional, I think some conventionally trained physicians find it easy to dismiss the idea of alternative medicine because they are not trained in it. Therefore, they can't advise a course of treatment. If you feel you must lie or withhold information to keep your doctor happy, perhaps you ought to think about finding another doctor.

Make simple changes. It never fails to impress me that often the simplest treatments offer the most amazing results. Examples of simple treatments include drinking a few cups of tea a day or applying salve two or three times a day. Frequently, these simple remedies have been successful when antibiotics, steroids, and other drugs have failed to do the job.

In my family, herbal medicine has meant the end to skin and sinus issues. Overall, we are pretty healthy. In my practice, I work with children who suffer from chronic issues like acne, arthritis, boils, eczema, menstrual difficulties, and migraines, to name just a few. I find that in most cases a simple change of diet and a simple herbal treatment not only offer dramatic change but also completely alleviate the issue.

Know where to buy herbs and herbal products. Most parents who call me with questions about an herbal remedy have purchased the product from a company for which herbs are a sideline and not a core business. Choose a company that specializes in herbs. Purchase herbal products at a health-food store, natural-food store, or an herbal apothecary. If you make your own herbal remedies, you will use fresh or dried herbs. Dried herbs can usually be purchased in bulk in natural- or health-food stores.

Buy organic products and organically grown herbs whenever possible. Using chemical-free herbs is as important as eating chemical-free foods. Supporting organic herb farming helps to promote sustainability, reduces land and water pollution, and is safer not only for our children but also for farmers and farm workers.

Read the label. When you purchase a prepared herbal medicine for your child, make sure it is formulated for children and labeled as such. If it is not—and most herbal remedies are made for adults—read the label to see of there is a children's dosage guideline. If not, you will have to adjust the dosage for your child (see Dosage Guidelines, page 64).

In addition, be certain the herb in the preparation is actually the herb you are looking for by checking the Latin genus and species name (for example, *Rubus idaeus*).

Follow dosing instructions. I know this sounds simple and perhaps even condescending, but it is rule number one. I've had a lot of phone calls from parents who are having problems with a remedy and, after much questioning and discussion, I've learned they simply aren't following the manufacturer's instructions.

Herbal products, even if they're for the same illness, contain different amounts of herbs and compounds, so the remedy you purchase may call for a different dosage than the one a friend purchased for her kids. Likewise, don't assume the dosage instructions will be the same if you buy a similar product the next time your child needs a remedy. Knowing the correct dosage can mean the difference between healing your child safely and effectively or enduring a lingering illness.

Respect that "natural" does not necessarily equal "safe." Do not assume that herbs can be used with impunity because they are natural, which only means "from nature." Plants "from nature" can contain poisons, or they can contain soothing and healing compounds. The use of herbal medicines can be extremely safe and beneficial. Most herbals, when used properly, have few side effects and work gently and effectively to prevent or heal illness. As with all medicines, there are guidelines that need to be understood and followed to ensure their effectiveness and safety.

Remember that herbs are not drugs. The most common mistake people make when using herbal remedies is treating them as if they are drugs. Although they have constituents like drugs and can treat illnesses as drugs do, herbs are *not* drugs. They are plants; herbal medicine is plant medicine. I use the word "drugs" to refer to synthetic or pharmaceutical preparations. A drug is a chemical substance, often prescribed by a medical provider, that is used in the diagnosis, treatment, or prevention of a condition or disease.

Unlike drugs, herbs have gentle—but effective—action. Herbalists don't administer remedies at the highest possible dose as a doctor might do with a prescription drug. Although some herbal treatments work swiftly, a parent shouldn't expect dramatic changes shortly after administering herbal remedies like she might after giving her child a prescription drug. Herbs work well, but they may take a little longer to do the job.

Overall, herbal remedies are more effective than drugs. However, keep in mind that although many herbal teas are safe for daily use over time, stronger forms of herbs, such as extracts, should not be used for more than brief periods without supervision by a trained herbalist or medical professional.

Listen to your child. You know your child better than anyone, including your doctor or a professional herbalist. Discontinue a remedy immediately if you think it's disagreeing with your child in some way, or if you think it's causing additional or undesirable symptoms. I do not subscribe to the "healing crisis" theory that sometimes the patient has to get worse before he gets better. A child should *not* get worse before he gets better. If he does get sicker, consult your doctor or health-care practitioner right away.

Follow the guidelines embodied in the acronym CARE:

Caution: Ask yourself if your child really needs a remedy. Perhaps his body can recover with rest and good food. If you believe your child needs a remedy, pay close attention to his symptoms and do more research to find a more appropriate remedy. Perhaps there is a gentler medicine.

Assessment: I like to say look, listen, and even smell your child. What does your child's body and actions "say" about the illness? Even if your child is too young to express herself, she can tell you how she's feeling and what hurts in other ways. Is she displaying different behavior? Is her skin clammy, dry, slick, or sweaty? Does she smell different? Often, parents know their child is ill by body smell, breath smell, feces odor, and urine odor. These clues can help you identify an illness and select a remedy.

Respect: Know what herbal remedy you're using and why *before* you give it to your child. I often hear parents say that they heard about a remedy from a friend, a clerk at a shop, or from someone who was selling it online. You don't show respect for your child by blindly offering him a remedy because you heard from somewhere that it *might* work.

Education: I can't stress this enough, and I'm sure I sound like a broken record, but education is key for all parents who are considering using herbal remedies for their kids. Yes, herbs *are* natural and therefore considered safe, but only if you know how to use them. If you're not sure, consult a trained herbalist or other health-care practitioner who is knowledgeable about herbal medicine, such as an acupuncturist, Chinese medicine doctor, homeopath, or naturopath.

When to Call a Doctor

Do not use the advice in this book or any of the resources listed as a replacement for proper medical care, especially in an emergency.

Seek medical care immediately if your child

- appears to be in a comalike state
- doesn't or won't make eye contact with you
- is lethargic, limp, or difficult to awaken
- is too sick to fuss or complain
- lies or sits lifelessly
- won't speak or moans incoherently
- won't walk or sit up.

Call a doctor if your child

- appears sick and is younger than two months of age
- becomes delirious or exhibits serious confusion, slurred speech, or the inability to perform simple motor functions
- complains of a stiff neck (a warning sign of meningitis)
- has a fever higher than 104 degrees Fahrenheit at any age
- has a fever higher than 100.5 degrees Fahrenheit at three month of age or younger
- has a rash that looks like bruising
- has balance and coordination problems
- has convulsions or seizures
- has difficulty breathing, has a blue tinge to the skin, makes rasping sounds (possibly after inhaling a foreign object), or sucks in air, making a hollow in the chest and thrusting the chin forward
- has ingested poison (call 911 or a poison control center)
- is dehydrated, is not urinating or has dark urine, has sunken eyes, and cries without tears (an infant's fontanel will be sunken)
- is three years of age or older and is drooling, has a high fever, and a muffled voice.

Don't be afraid to call a doctor if you are just plain worried.

Combining Herbs Safely with Other Medications

Combining herbal remedies with drugs can be dangerous. If your child is on medication, make sure you research each herb's interactions with that particular drug before giving the herb to your child. For instance, if your child takes a selective serotonin reuptake inhibitor, such as Prozac or Paxil, for the treatment of depression, he should not be given St. John's wort. Another problematic combination is garlic capsules and some diabetes medications, which can cause a dangerous decrease in blood sugar levels when taken together.

Most drug–herb interaction problems occur with adult medications and herbs, especially ones that affect blood pressure and clotting factors.

FINDING AN HERBALIST

If you're unsure which herbal course to take, if your child has health issues that are confounding the situation for you, or if you just want to be sure you're on the right track, my best advice is to consult an herbalist or an herbal practitioner.

Herbalists generally have two to eight years of traditional education and hands-on training in addition to about five years of some type of college education. The belief that herbalists are uninformed and uneducated is a misconception. Most train formally at education centers, schools, and colleges, or participate in apprenticeships or distance-learning programs. They are trained to use herbs, of course, but they also know how and when to add nutrition therapy. They will also recommend other alternatives, such as acupuncture or homeopathy, if they think it's needed.

Finding an herbalist may be as easy as looking in the phone book or on the Internet. You also can request a referral from an acupuncturist, a chiropractor, a doula, a massage therapist, a midwife, a naturopath, or any professional in complementary and alternative medicine.

Here are some tips for finding a good herbalist:

Ask a doctor. If your doctor is unaccepting or unsupportive of your decision to use herbs for your child's illnesses, you may want to find another doctor. Contact a doctor of Chinese medicine or a practitioner of homeopathic medicine. They routinely prescribe medicinal herbs for their patients and may be able to recommend an herbalist.

Ask your friends. Other parents who have used herbal medicines with their own children may be able to make a recommendation.

Contact the American Herbalist Guild. (See Herb Associations, page 195.) An herbalist who is a member will be guaranteed to have a certain level of education and training. However, some competent and qualified herbalists disagree with the guild's certification process and are not members. In addition, herbalists who run schools or other training programs may not be listed because they are educators and do not see clients as their primary business. Just because an herbalist is not a member of the American Herbalist Guild does not necessarily mean he or she is not a competent herbalist.

Contact a local or regional herbal medicine school. (See Herbalism Schools, page 195.) Your local alternative newspaper or natural-food store might provide information about herbal schools. Also, see www.naturalhealers.com.

Talk to the staff at your natural-food store. They may be able to offer suggestions or referrals to local herbal practitioners. However, do not rely on the employees for medical advice unless, of course, they are herbalists. Many are not qualified and may merely repeat information given to them by the companies whose products are sold in the store. While this advice may not necessarily be incorrect, it cannot be considered competent medical advice.

Questions to Ask an Herbalist

As you would do with any health-care practitioner, ask an herbalist about her education, experience, fees, specialties, and so on. Feel free to ask for her resume or request references. Call the school she attended to see if she graduated from the program. This is done routinely, so don't feel shy about doing this.

It's important to check up on someone who will be taking your child's health into her hands, particularly since, in the United States, there are few if any regulations or requirements about who can call herself an herbalist. Because anyone can hang out a shingle, parents must choose an herbalist with care. An informed choice will always be the best choice.

It's also important to ask whether an herbalist has worked with children and, if so, for how long. In my area, a husband and wife herbalist team set themselves up as ADHD experts, but admitted during a presentation that they'd treated only one child with their herbal protocol. Of course, a remedy's effectiveness cannot be based solely on one client's outcome.

Don't be rude when asking questions, but don't dismiss any lingering doubts either. If the herbalist will not answer a question, gets defensive, is evasive, or responds with a question, she may not be the right practitioner for you. If an herbalist bases your child's treatment on a set product line or an all-encompassing remedy, you may want to find another practitioner. Herbalism is not a product-specific practice.

You can buy a remedy in a store at any time, but when you decide to consult an herbalist, you are doing so to get something more: a remedy that is compounded for the specific needs of your child. Your provider is your choice. You can change or leave at any time.

HERBAL STYLES

Herbal practices can vary from country to country, state to state, city to city, and herbalist to herbalist. Each herbal practitioner is unique, offering care and healing from an individual perspective and his or her chosen style of practice. You may also find that the herbalist you consult uses a variety of styles and resources. Following are the general styles of herbal practice:

Ayurveda

Ayurveda is an ancient system of health care that originated in India more than 4,000 years ago. Today, it is used daily by millions of people there, as well as in Sri Lanka and Nepal. Indirectly, it has also influenced Chinese and Tibetan medicine.

Ayurveda is based on the theory that illness results when the life force, or *prana*, of the body is out of balance. Ayurvedic doctors and practitioners heal illness by balancing characteristics of the prana, called *doshas*. To balance the doshas, ayurvedic doctors suggest specific herbs and dietary changes.

The Eclectics

Eclectic herbalism has its roots in a group of American medical doctors who practiced from the mid-1800s through the 1930s and primarily used botanical medicines to treat their patients. The Eclectics were traditionally trained medical doctors who broke away from medical practices of their day, such as blood letting and purges with calomel and other mercury-based remedies. The Eclectics had a philosophy of "alignment with nature," and they embraced wisdom and concepts from other schools of thought as well.

Eclectic physicians numbered in the thousands. They published an extensive number of books and journals and cared for millions of patients for almost one hundred years. The Eclectic movement was a powerful medical body until the formation of the American Medical Association (AMA), which preferred pharmaceutical medicines over herbal remedies. After the formation of the AMA, it became increasingly hard to fund and run Eclectic medical schools.

The tremendously rapid growth of allopathic medicine (the common medical practice we know today) was funded by millions of dollars from institutions such as the Rockefeller and Carnegie foundations, leading to the demise of the Eclectics in the early 1900s. The knowledge they developed, however, never lost favor among herbalists and naturopathic physicians worldwide.

Eclectics kept extensive materia medicas that still offer many gems of relevant and effective herbal information. Modern eclectic herbalists also use Native American traditions in herbalism and botanical research.

Folk Herbalism

Throughout the world, folk herbalism combines regional and traditional practices. In the United States, it combines the traditions of Native Americans, the early colonists, and herbalists in Appalachia. Folk herbalism often combines dream interpretation with cultural beliefs and practices. Folk medicine is recorded in the oral tradition, and mainstream medical practitioners do not generally respect it.

Folk herbalists can be found all over the world. In more remote areas, a folk herbalist may be a community's primary health-care provider. Although these practitioners have been ridiculed in herbal, historical, and medical writings, a majority of herbal remedies and pharmaceutical drugs have their roots in the "cures" of the folk herbalists.

Naturopathic Medicine

Naturopathic medicine incorporates traditional natural therapies with modern scientific medical diagnoses and Western medical standards of care. Naturopathic physicians prescribe herbs and use other healing modalities, such as acupuncture, clinical nutrition, homeopathy, hydrotherapy, naturopathic manipulative therapy, and traditional Chinese medicine (TCM). Naturopathic medicine is growing in popularity and is increasingly accepted by insurance companies and mainstream Western medicine.

In the United States, there are only a few accredited schools of naturopathy. Just as anyone who thinks he knows herbal medicine can hang out a shingle, so can anyone who believes he can practice naturopathy. A degree in naturopathy cannot be obtained via distance learning, so make sure the naturopath you are interviewing has a degree from an accredited school. (While someone who is self-educated or who has done coursework at home via a correspondence school may have some good advice, he has not undergone naturopathic medical education and study in the basic and clinical sciences, nor completed a clinical internship.) In particular, beware of individuals who call themselves "traditional naturopaths."

Traditional Chinese Medicine

Traditional Chinese medicine, often referred to as TCM, is thousands of years old. The system is based on the belief that illness results when there is a blockage or improper flow of *qi,* the life force or energy, through the body. Qi is restored by balancing the opposing forces of *yin* and *yang* with various tools, such as acupuncture, diet, herbs, and massage.

With a history of two to three thousand years, TCM has become a unique system with which to diagnose and treat illness. The TCM approach is fundamentally different from that of Western medicine. In TCM, the understanding of the human body is based on the holistic understanding of the universe as described in Taoism, and the treatment of illness is based primarily on the diagnosis and differentiation of syndromes. As a healing system, TCM is composed of adjunct components, such as acupuncture, cupping, massage, and the application of heat to the skin using burning herbs (a process known as moxibustion).

Herbal medicines have been used in China for centuries, and their use has been supported by a long and rich history of development and research. Chinese herbal medicine is unique in that the diagnosis and treatments are based on the theories of traditional Chinese medicine. TCM practitioners note signs and symptoms, such as the look of the tongue and the "reading" of the pulse, to make diagnoses. In the case of the common cold, for instance, a patient may be diagnosed as having "wind-cold invasion," and herbs that dispel wind and warm the body would probably be suggested.

Western Herbalism

Western herbalism has its roots in the indigenous cultures of North and South America, including Native Americans, Mexican Indians, and Inuit, and from early American settlers, including people from Appalachia, the southern United States, and New England.

Western herbalism uses local and regional plants. A Western herbalist in rural Vermont may draw on regional herbal practices and practices from French Canadian ancestors. Similarly, a California herbalist might also embrace Mexican remedies, and an herbalist in North Carolina might include Appalachian heritage remedies.

Western herbalism is based on the herbalists' clinical experience and traditional knowledge of medicinal plant remedies as preserved by oral tradition and in written records over thousands of years. To me, Western herbalism is *my* people's medicine. I can use traditions from my ancestors and remedies from my life, my cupboards, and my yard to heal my family and myself.

Western herbalism is somewhat like the much older folk system but is more structured than, say, traditional Chinese medicine because it relies on the synergistic and curative properties of the plant to treat symptoms and disease and maintain health. Whereas Chinese medicine encompasses herbalism, acupuncture, dietary therapy, and massage, Western herbalists look to traditional folk practices, historical uses of herbs, and modern science to diagnose and prescribe.

The Herbal Medicine Chest: Commonly Used Herbs

When purchasing herbs—whether as a ready-made remedy from a natural-food store or as dried plants from a bulk supplier—be certain you have properly identified the ones you need. The only way to know for sure is to look for the Latin genus and species name. A folk name or a common name, such as "coneflower" or "snakeroot," can vary from region to region and may not indicate the plant you think it does.

Accurate plant identification is paramount when preparing and using herbal remedies. This is especially important when buying dried herbs in bulk because dried herbs all look pretty much the same. Labels should include the herb's common name, botanical or Latin name, date of harvest, and the name of the grower, manufacturer, or packager. Here is an example:

In addition, details should be provided about the herb's place of origin, weight, and how it was grown (conventionally, organically, or wildcrafted, meaning harvested from a natural or wild habitat). For my herbal remedies, I provide the following information:

- the common name
- the Latin name
- the herb's curing abilities
- conditions the herb is prescribed for
- cautions about using the herb
- contraindications for that particular herb

Common name: Red Raspberry Leaf

Latin genus and species name: Rubus idaeus

Date of harvest: August 20, 2010

Name of the grower, manufacturer, or packager: XYZ Herb Company

THE LANGUAGE OF HERBAL MEDICINE

Herbalists use specialized terms to define different types of herbal preparations. One important distinction is whether an herb is taken internally or orally, such as an herbal tea or tonic, or used externally, such as a compress or liniment.

Herbal Preparations

This book contains instructions for preparing many types of herbal preparations. These are described in detail in chapter 5. Following is a brief overview that can be helpful as you read chapters 2, 3, and 4.

Compress. A compress is used externally to accelerate the healing process. It is made by soaking a piece of cloth in a decoction or infusion and applying it either hot or cold to the affected area.

Decoction. A decoction is the concentrated liquor that results after heating or boiling down plant parts such as bark, nuts, or roots. Decoctions are used to make teas and are ingredients in compresses and liniments.

Extract. An extract is a remedy that contains the active ingredient(s) of an herb in a concentrated form. The herb is usually extracted by soaking it for a long period in alcohol or pure vegetable glycerin.

Essential oil. Essential oils are aromatic and healing substances that have been distilled from plants. They contain highly concentrated and potent compounds.

Infusion. An infusion is a remedy made by soaking plant parts or dried herbs in a liquid. Herbal tea is the most well-known and popular herbal infusion. Infused oils make it easy to administer an herb's healing compounds.

Liniment. A liniment is an herbal extraction in a liquid, such as alcohol, oil, or vinegar, that is rubbed into the skin to treat arthritis, inflammations, sore muscles, and strains.

Lozenge. A lozenge, or pastille, is a small bit of medicine designed to be held in the mouth and dissolved slowly. Lozenges are used to help alleviate sore throats, calm coughs, freshen breath, and aid digestion.

Plaster. A plaster is similar to a poultice but is typically made of dried herbs. Plasters are used externally for treating muscle pains and strains and other general aches and pains. They should not be used on open wounds or damaged or irritated skin. They also should not be used on children younger than two years of age.

Poultice. A poultice is similar to a compress except that fresh plant parts are used. Poultices are considered more "active" than compresses. They are used externally to stimulate circulation, ease aches and pains, or draw impurities from the body through the skin; therefore, they need to remain in place for a few hours at a time.

Salve. A salve is a cream or emollient used on the skin to provide protection while carrying medicinal benefits.

Syrup. A syrup is a thick solution of sugar and water that is flavored or medicated, such as a cough syrup.

Tincture. A tincture is traditionally a diluted extract. The terms "extract" and "tincture" are often interchanged and misused these days.

Tonic. A tonic is an herb (or herbal blend) that strengthens and tones the entire body or specific organs through nutritional support.

Actions of Herbal Remedies

Herbalists use specialized terms to define the many different effects of herbal remedies. More than one of the following descriptors can apply to a given herb:

Adaptogen. Adaptogenic herbs heighten resistance and endurance to help the body resist biological, chemical, and physical stresses and adapt to extraordinary challenges.

Anodyne or analgesic. Anodynes, also called analgesics, work internally or externally to reduce pain.

Antibacterial. Antibacterials inhibit the growth of bacteria.

Anti-inflammatory. Anti-inflammatories help the body combat inflammation.

Antimicrobial. Antimicrobials help the body's immune system destroy or resist disease-causing microorganisms.

Antiseptic. Antiseptics prevent and counteract inflammation and infection.

Antispasmodic. Antispasmodics prevent or ease spasms and cramps.

Aromatic. Aromatics have strong and often pleasant odors, and can stimulate the digestive juices.

Astringent. Astringents contract, tighten, and strengthen tissue and can reduce secretions and discharges.

Carminative. Carminatives are rich in volatile aromatic oils and expel gas from the stomach and bowels, supporting peristalsis and healthy digestion.

Cathartic. In large doses, cathartics purge the bowels and stimulate glandular secretions.

Cholagogue. Cholagogues stimulate secretion of bile from the gallbladder. They can also have a laxative effect.

Choleretic. Choleretics increase the production of bile in the liver.

Demulcent. Demulcents coat the throat and other mucous membranes to relieve irritation and inflammation, such as a sore throat, and help stop coughing.

Diaphoretic. Diaphoretics stimulate perspiration and elimination through the skin.

Diuretic. Diuretics increase urinary output.

Emmenagogue. Emmenagogues stimulate and normalize menstruation and the menstrual cycle.

Expectorant. Expectorants help the respiratory system to expel excess mucus.

Hypotensive. Hypotensives can reduce elevated blood pressure.

Laxative. Laxatives promote bowel movements and relieve constipation.

Nervine. Nervines strengthen, tone, and nourish the nervous system, easing anxiety and stress.

Pectoral. Pectorals have a general strengthening and healing effect on the respiratory system.

Secretolytic. Secretolytics loosen hardened or impacted mucus.

Sedative. Sedatives soothe the central nervous system, relieving anxiety and causing sleepiness.

Spasmolytic. Spasmolytics prevent or relieve spasms.

Stimulant. Stimulants enliven and quicken physiological functions.

Vulnerary. Vulneraries have wound-healing capabilities.

HERBS USED IN REMEDIES FOR CHILDREN

Alfalfa (*Medicago sativa*)

Alfalfa is prescribed for overall nutrition and health. It is a gentle diuretic that also promotes appetite, so it is especially good for children who are lethargic or who have a weak constitution and can't gain weight. Alfalfa may also be beneficial for reducing cholesterol levels. It is high in vitamins, minerals, and antioxidants, so I often include it in children's remedies for its nourishing benefits.

CAUTIONS: Children should be given alfalfa only as an infusion and not in tablet form.

CONTRAINDICATIONS: None known.

Aloe vera (*Aloe barbadensis*)

Aloe vera has been in recorded use for more than five thousand years, which is a pretty good lifespan for a remedy. It has impressive skin-healing abilities, especially on burned or sunburned skin, due to its high content of a type of polysaccharide that stimulates skin growth and repair. Aloe vera is also used to treat digestive conditions. (However, I do not recommend that it be used to treat constipation in young children without the advice of a doctor, health-care practitioner, or an herbalist. Overuse can be dangerous.)

CONTRAINDICATIONS: None for topical use.

American cranesbill (*Geranium maculatum*)

A powerful astringent, American cranesbill contains compounds that cause mucous membranes to constrict, making it effective against cholera, diarrhea, dysentery, hemorrhage, and nosebleeds. It is used internally for intestinal bleeding and for reducing inflammation of the mucous membranes. It is also found in remedies that help to heal mouth sores, sore throats, and bleeding gums. In addition, it is a valuable treatment for hemorrhoids.

CONTRAINDICATIONS: Cranesbill is not recommended for long-term use. Excessive use may cause liver damage.

Angelica (*Angelica archangelica*)

This form of angelica is most often used to stimulate appetite and relieve flatulence and other gastrointestinal spasms. Because of its expectorant properties, it is also used in remedies for urinary tract infections and coughs. There's a long history of using angelica for coughs in Europe, where it is given in candied form to children with colds. Angelica is also added to cough medicines.

CONTRAINDICATIONS: Angelica contains furanocoumarins, a chemical compound produced by plants that can sensitize the skin to sunlight and cause sunburn. Keep your children out of the sun if they've taken a remedy containing this herb.

Anise (*Pimpinella anisum*)

Anise is a carminative and pectoral herb. For hundreds of years, it has been used for lung conditions and coughs, particularly harsh, dry coughs. Anise is a popular ingredient in lozenges. The seeds are often used in remedies for colic and to ease gas and indigestion. In addition, anise is an antimicrobial, antispasmodic, and expectorant.

CONTRAINDICATIONS: Occasional allergic reactions have been reported.

Arnica (*Arnica montana*)

When applied externally, infused oil of arnica or homeopathic arnica tincture or ointment stimulates the peripheral blood supply and improves circulation, making it one of the best herbal remedies for bruises, sprains, and strains. It also has a soothing effect on achy muscles. As the mother of two active boys, I never go out of the house without arnica oil. I've seen this herbal oil work many times and am always impressed by its dramatic action. Because it is an anti-inflammatory and a vulnerary, arnica is excellent for treating damaged and bruised areas.

CAUTIONS: Arnica herb is never to be taken internally. Pure arnica essential oil can be toxic. Instead, use only infused oil or homeopathic arnica products. (See Additional Cautions, page 58.)

CONTRAINDICATIONS: Never use arnica oil on broken skin.

Astragalus (Astragalus membranaceus)

Astragalus is quite the wonder herb. It increases the activity of natural killer cells, strengthening the immune system. It scavenges pathogenic bacteria, such as diphtheria, pneumonia, and tuberculosis, and those that cause foodborne illnesses. And it contains powerful antioxidants that fight free radicals, which can damage cells. It is included in remedies that fight cancer, colds, diabetes, heart disease, high blood pressure, liver diseases, and upper respiratory infections.

Astragalus also has antibacterial and anti-inflammatory properties, and is sometimes used topically for wounds. In addition, studies have shown that astragalus has antiviral properties. As an adaptogen, astragalus helps normalize bodily systems.

CAUTIONS: Astragalus can be effective against fever, but only if it is used when the fever is first noticed. Don't give astragalus for a lingering fever. "Loco weed," as astragalus is known in some parts of the United States, is a different species from *Astragalus membranaceus*. It has different effects from the herb that is referred to in this book. Do not substitute loco weed for *Astragalus membranaceus*.

CONTRAINDICATIONS: Do not give your child astragalus without consulting your doctor if your child is taking immune-suppressing drugs such as corticosteroids and cyclophosphamide, which is used in chemotherapy and to reduce rejection in transplant recipients.

Basil (Ocimum basilicum)

As a medicinal herb, basil is often referred to as part of herb royalty—its name may have been derived from the Greek *basileus*, which means "king" or "royal." Basil has a rich and varied history; cultures all over the world know and respect its healing powers. Basil is used for coughs, exhaustion, flu, migraines, nausea, sore muscles, stress relief, and stomach cramps.

Bergamot (*Citrus aurantium, C. bergamia*)

With active ingredients that are antibiotic, antiseptic, antispasmodic, and calmative, bergamot essential oil just about does it all. It's included in remedies for anxiety, depression, and pain. It's also useful for appetite loss and skin issues, such as abscesses, boils, cold sores, itching, and psoriasis. Used in a diffuser, bergamot helps improve seasonal affective disorder and alleviate stress.

CONTRAINDICATIONS: Bergamot should not be taken orally. It can cause phototoxicity. Keep your children out of direct sun for twenty-four hours after giving bergamot.

Black walnut (*Juglans nigra*)

Black walnut is a strong antifungal that is helpful for healing skin conditions, such as eczema, herpes, and shingles, and fighting fungal infections, such as athlete's foot and jock itch. It is also used in remedies for intestinal parasites.

CONTRAINDICATIONS: Children with walnut allergy should not be given black walnut.

Blackberry leaf (*Rubus fruticosus*)

Blackberry leaf tea has long been used to treat diarrhea because of its astringent compounds. It can also be used to treat insect bites. Topically, as a compress or poultice, it helps heal wounds and burns; as a gargle, it helps heal inflamed gums, mouth ulcers, and sore throats.

CAUTIONS: Because it is strong and highly astringent, blackberry leaf should only be prescribed to children older than two years of age and used only as a tea for a day or two. (It can cause constipation or diarrhea if used longer than that.) Seek alternative treatment if there's no change in your child's health in that time.

Boneset (*Eupatorium perfoliatum*)

Boneset contains polysaccharides that have been shown to stimulate the immune system, making it a good choice in remedies for bacterial infections, colds, coughs, and flu. Used as a tonic for the gastric system, it increases appetite and improves digestion.

CAUTIONS: Medical literature suggests that boneset use should be limited to one week. It should not be used for long periods of time because its high alkaloid content can prove toxic. In my opinion, however, no direct evidence exists for this warning.

Burdock (*Arctium lappa*)

When I did a plant spirit medicine workshop a few years ago, this was the herb that spoke to me. I found myself delving into its uses and wonders for a long time. This herb is a powerhouse.

Burdock is used to clear the skin and is a valuable remedy for the treatment of skin conditions that result in dry and scaly skin, including bruises, burns, dandruff, eczema, and psoriasis. (European practitioners use it in treatments for rheumatic disorders, especially when psoriasis is present.) Burdock is an important ingredient in remedies for anorexia nervosa, cystitis, digestion, herpes, joint swelling, kidney problems, poor appetite, sore joints, ulcers, and wound healing.

Burdock root is used to cleanse the liver and fortify the blood. Tincture stimulates the immune system and restores liver and gallbladder function.

CONTRAINDICATIONS: Contact with the plant may cause an allergic reaction on the skin.

Calendula (*Calendula officinalis*)

Calendula's powers to regenerate the skin are due to the flower's high carotenoid, flavonoid, and saponin content. Studies have shown that these compounds support wound healing and skin repair; they also have anti-inflammatory properties. Calendula products are used for treating chapped and cracked skin, diaper rash, eczema, and skin rashes. Calendula is also a good treatment for cuts and scrapes, cradle cap, mild burns, and sore muscles.

CONTRAINDICATIONS: Calendula should not be given internally to children unless prescribed by a professional (see page 61.)

Camphor (*Cinnamomum camphora*)

Camphor is a well-known ingredient in rubs, salves, and other topical applications. In a chest rub, it helps break up chest mucus and relieves congestion; in a body rub, it eases sore joints and muscles. In steam inhalation—safe only for children six years of age and older—camphor clears and helps release the mucus of colds and flu.

CONTRAINDICATIONS: Camphor is strong and powerful; it should not be used internally. External application can cause skin irritation or eczema. Inhalation can be dangerous; follow directions carefully.

Caraway (*Carum carvi*)

Caraway is an ingredient in remedies that relieve gas and intestinal colic, stimulate the appetite, relieve sore throat and laryngitis, and treat bronchitis and asthma.

Cardamom (*Elettaria cardamomum*)

Many people associate this herb with Indian cuisine and chai, but it is also a great medicinal to have in your kitchen and your herbal medicine chest. I prescribe cardamom for infections and digestive disorders, particularly for relieving gas. Cardamom is also good for relieving sore gums and toothaches. Because it tastes great, it's easy to get little ones to drink cardamom.

Catnip (*Nepeta cataria*)

Catnip is another herb with incredibly diverse uses. It's an ingredient in remedies for everything from upset stomach and digestive distress to chronic bronchitis, diarrhea, and fever. The herb is also strongly antifungal and a bactericide for staphylococci. In addition, it is a close chemical relative of a number of insect repellents that affect mosquitoes and termites. Catnip has long been used in remedies for anxiety, colic, headaches, insomnia, and toothaches, and in liniments for muscle aches.

Chamomile (*Matricaria recutita*)

Chamomile is one of the most popular herbs and often one of the first most people try. (If you've ever had a cup of Sleepytime tea from Celestial Seasonings, you've had chamomile.) Chamomile is known for its sedating effects and its anti-inflammatory properties. You will find it in products for conditions as diverse as canker sores, colic, eczema, indigestion, sore gums, and teething.

CAUTIONS: Children with hay fever and other upper respiratory allergies can also be allergic to chamomile.

Chaparral (*Larrea tridentata*)

Chaparral is a strong-acting herb, so I never use it in internal remedies for infants or young children. However, when used externally, chaparral works well in compresses, lotions, and salves to treat skin conditions, such as chicken pox, cold sores, contact dermatitis, eczema, psoriasis, and shingles. I have also successfully used chaparral compresses on children with weepy and discolored psoriasis.

CONTRAINDICATIONS: Give chaparral remedies to children only on the recommendation of a doctor, health-care practitioner, or herbalist. Although chaparral has a long history of use, its safety for internal use is still in question. Used topically, it is generally considered safe.

Chickweed (*Stellaria media*)

Chickweed is commonly used in topical remedies for itching and other skin irritations, such as eczema and psoriasis, and to speed the healing of cuts and wounds. It's also used internally for anxiety-induced stomachaches and for eczema, rheumatism, sore muscles and joints, sore throats, ulcers, and urinary problems. Chickweed is used in poultices and compresses to ease rheumatic pain and treat boils, abscesses, and hemorrhoids. Chickweed poultices are also used to draw out splinters and insect stingers. As an extract, it can be used topically to treat warts. An infusion may be added to bath water to soothe inflamed skin.

Cinnamon (*Cinnamomum spp.*)

Yes, this is the same cinnamon you have on your kitchen spice shelf; it can be purchased almost everywhere. Cinnamon is known for its ability to warm the body and aid digestion, so it's great for soothing upset tummies. It can also boost vitality in kids who tend to contract flu easily, and it is helpful in treating diarrhea that is associated with stress. As a tea it is antibacterial, antiseptic, antispasmodic, and carminative, all of which are beneficial in treating coughs. It can be used as a component in decoctions, syrups, and tinctures for the flavor and excellent healing benefits it offers. The herb and essential oil have much different properties, so research the essential oil before using.

CONTRAINDICATIONS: Use with care. Doses exceeding two grams, or one-half teaspoon to one teaspoon of ground cinnamon, have been shown to be narcotic and may cause convulsions, delirium, hallucinations, and even death in adults. Treatment with cinnamon is inadvisable for people with a cinnamon allergy. (A sprinkle of cinnamon or a small amount in or on food is generally, of course, not an issue.) Essential oil of cinnamon is very strong and must be diluted before using topically.

Clary sage (*Salvia sclarea*)

Clary sage is found in herbal remedies for asthma, coughing, intestinal gas, sore throat, whooping cough, and all types of skin conditions. As an essential oil massaged on the abdomen, it can lessen gas pains. It can also be massaged into painful joints or hurting muscles. (The essential oil needs to be diluted when applied to skin.) In the shower, it becomes steam inhalation therapy for respiratory problems, such as asthma, coughing, sore throat, and whooping cough, and as a stress and anxiety reliever. Clary sage is often prescribed for emotional issues, including paranoia.

Cleavers (*Galium aparine*)

Cleavers is known as a great tonic for the lymph system, making it quick and effective in the treatment of tonsillitis (use the tea as a gargle) and swollen lymph glands. Taken internally as a tincture or a tea, cleavers helps heal eczema, cystitis, and psoriasis. It also helps stop bed-wetting.

CONTRAINDICATIONS: Cleavers is a strong diuretic, so do not give it to a child who is already taking diuretics. Children who have diabetes probably should not use cleavers, because it may overstimulate the adrenal glands and reduce the action of insulin.

Cloves (*Eugenia caryophyllata*)

Clove is an antispasmodic and antibacterial herb, and its use has been documented for more than one thousand years. Clove oil, also called clove bud oil, can be derived from the bud, the leaf, or the stem; it has been used for centuries to relieve the pain of muscle aches and, most famously, toothaches. To this day, dentists use clove oil to kill nerve pain when filling cavities and performing root canals. Clove tea is also good for stomachaches and other digestive upsets; however, clove is high in flavorful essential oils, so it's often too strong for a child's palate. That's why you'll usually find cloves mixed with other herbs in children's remedies.

CAUTIONS: Do not give the essential oil for internal use.

Coltsfoot (*Tussilago farfara*)

Coltsfoot has been used medicinally as a cough suppressant for centuries. Traditionally, it has been given for acute breathing disorders, bronchitis, dry coughs, and sore throats. Currently, the German government commission on herbs recommends coltsfoot tea as a remedy for a hoarse, dry cough with thick mucus and sore throat. I also find it helps children with bronchial issues and laryngitis.

CONTRAINDICATIONS: Do not give coltsfoot to children with heart or blood pressure problems without consulting a doctor or health-care practitioner. Use coltsfoot remedies carefully.

Comfrey (*Symphytum officinale*)

Comfrey cools down inflamed skin and helps heal rashes and other skin problems, including burns and diaper rash. It is also said to speed the healing of broken bones and sprains. Comfrey's healing capabilities are attributed to a compound called allantoin, which has soothing, anti-irritating, and antiaging properties. The herb is a well-known vulnerary, or wound healer, but its use is controversial.

CAUTIONS: Britain banned the internal use of comfrey in 1992 because it contains certain alkaloids that can damage the liver. Therefore, comfrey should only be used externally, and only the leaves of the plant should be used when making remedies. (See Additional Cautions, page 58.)

Cramp bark (*Viburnum opulus*)

As its name suggests, cramp bark is a muscle relaxant.

CONTRAINDICATIONS: Because cramp bark, like aspirin, contains salicin, children who are allergic to aspirin may also be allergic to cramp bark. Cramp bark should not be given to children who are taking blood-thinning medications. It may also lower blood pressure or cause gastroenteritis.

Cypress (*Cupressus sempervirens*)

Cypress essential oil can be found in remedies for excessive perspiration, hemorrhoids, and varicose veins. In a diffuser, the oil can be used as a remedy for coughing.

Dandelion (*Taraxacum officinale*)

A powerful diuretic rich in unique compounds, dandelion has been used for years to reduce swelling and relieve muscle aches and pains. A known liver tonic, dandelion also has laxative effects and is beneficial for the kidneys and urinary tract.

CONTRAINDICATIONS: People who are allergic to latex may also be allergic to dandelion. Do not give dandelion to children who are suffering from bile duct obstruction, gallbladder or gastrointestinal inflammation, or intestinal blockage.

Dill (*Anethum graveolens*)

Dill, a great remedy for gas and colic, can be given to little ones as a tea. Just one teaspoon of the tea is a simple remedy for a colicky baby.

CAUTIONS: Dill seeds have been known to cause contact dermatitis.

CONTRAINDICATIONS: Dill has a high sodium content and may not be suitable for children on controlled sodium diets.

Echinacea (*Echinacea* spp.)

Echinacea contains antimicrobial, antiviral, and immune-stimulating compounds. It is well-known for its ability to fight bacterial and viral infections, particularly colds and flu. Echinacea is available in capsules, cough drops, tablets, teas, and tinctures.

CAUTIONS: Children who are allergic to chrysanthemums, marigolds, ragweed, and other members of the daisy family may also be allergic to echinacea. Children prone to allergies and asthma may also have adverse reactions to echinacea. Babies younger than two years of age should not be given echinacea in many circumstances. Short-term acute dosing is considered safe. (See Additional Cautions, page 58).

Elder (*Sambucus nigra*)

The berries and flowers from the elder tree have a multitude of uses. The flower is a diaphoretic used for treating colds, flu, and respiratory illnesses. One study showed that flu patients who took elderberry remedies healed in half the time of those who did not, most likely due to substances called Sambucus nigra agglutinins, which help prevent some strains of flu from infecting healthy cells. Studies currently being conducted have shown that elderberry may also be beneficial for patients with herpes, HIV, and other conditions that suppress the immune system. Elderberry is also used in poultices for pain and inflammation, and as a compress for sunburn and mild burns.

Children love the flavor of elderberries, so it's useful in many children's remedies. Even elderberry syrup on pancakes serves as a tonic for colds, flu, and other viral bugs.

CAUTIONS: Elderberry remedies are considered safe and relatively free of side effects when taken in the suggested doses (as indicated on product labels and the recipes in this book). The berries should not be eaten raw; uncooked berries may cause vomiting and diarrhea. Some constituents of the leaves, flowers, roots, and stems contain poisonous alkaloids. If your child is taking drugs that increase urination, consult your child's doctor or health-care practitioner before administering elder flower, since prolonged use or overuse may increase urination, resulting in the loss of potassium from the body.

Elecampane (*Inula helenium*)

Elecampane is an antiseptic, diaphoretic, and expectorant that is known for treating particularly irritating coughs. It is a respiratory tonic used to strengthen the overall system. Elecampane is a common ingredient in cough remedies and is used to treat chronic bronchitis and whooping cough. It's a gentle herb, which makes it perfect for kids.

CONTRAINDICATIONS: This herb may cause allergic reactions resulting in dermatitis. Large doses of this herb can cause diarrhea, spasms, vomiting, and symptoms of paralysis; follow usage and dosage instructions carefully.

Eucalyptus (*Eucalyptus globulus*)

Essential oil of eucalyptus is often used for treating arthritis, sore muscles, and respiratory ailments, such as congestion and coughing. In diffusers and vaporizers, it is used to help break up chest and nasal congestion.

CAUTIONS: Never use eucalyptus essential oil directly on the skin, even if it is diluted.

Eyebright (*Euphrasia officinalis*)

Eyebright is aptly named. It is used primarily in remedies (especially compresses) for conjunctivitis, eye infections and inflammations, and weeping eyes. The homeopathic version should be a mainstay in the medicine cabinet of any parent whose child suffers from hay fever and the related itchy, red, and swollen eyes. As a tea, eyebright helps treat sinusitis.

CONTRAINDICATIONS: Eyebright is usually safe when used topically.

Fennel (*Foeniculum vulgare*)

Fennel contains compounds that are anti-inflammatory, antispasmodic, and carminative. It makes an exceptionally good stomach and intestinal remedy because it relieves flatulence while at the same time stimulating digestion and appetite. Fennel is an integral part of many colic remedies.

CONTRAINDICATIONS: None are known for the herb, but the essential oil should not be used in children who are allergic to celery.

Frankincense (*Boswellia carteri*)

Essential oil of frankincense has a soothing and relaxing effect, so it's popular for relieving stress and anxiety. Its antiseptic and expectorant properties make it valuable in the treatment of asthma and bronchitis. As a compress, lotion, or massage oil, it is beneficial as a chest rub and skin antiseptic and for treating rheumatism and scars.

CONTRAINDICATIONS: It is generally considered safe.

Garlic (*Allium sativum*)

Garlic has been used in cooking and healing throughout the world for thousands of years. Its antimicrobial, antispasmodic, and hypotensive properties make it an important element in herbal remedies for digestive and respiratory conditions, athlete's foot, earaches, ringworm, and yeast infections. Garlic is inexpensive, readily available, and simple to use. Mince a clove or two and add it to butters and spreads, dips, main dishes, pastas, soups, salads and salad dressings, and vegetables—the list is almost endless. Garlic can also be taken as a tea, a tincture, or in a capsule.

CAUTIONS: Garlic should be discontinued as a supplement two to three weeks prior to any surgery because it thins the blood and could increase bleeding.

Geranium (*Pelargonium graveolens*)

Essential oil of geranium is an ingredient in remedies for head lice. It is also found in cosmetics and renowned for improving dull or oily skin.

CAUTIONS: Geranium can cause dermatitis in children with sensitive skin.

Ginger (*Zingiber officinale*)

Ginger is an herb common to many herbal traditions. It is well-known as a remedy for motion sickness and digestive upsets, such as colic in infants and gas, heartburn, and stomachaches in older children. It is also included in remedies for circulatory problems, coughing, and diarrhea. Like garlic, fresh ginger can be found in most supermarkets and natural-food stores, and it can be added to food or taken as a tea or tincture. Natural ginger ales are tasty and easy to administer to toddlers and children, as are candied or crystallized ginger, and ginger candy.

CAUTIONS: Large doses of this herb may irritate the mucous membranes of the stomach and bowel, so do not give more than the recommended dosage to anyone with stomach or bowel disorders. Laboratory research has shown that ginger can reduce platelet stickiness in blood, so consult your doctor or health-care practitioner before giving ginger to children who are taking blood thinners.

CONTRAINDICATIONS: Ginger is a cholagogue, so do not give ginger to anyone with gallstones.

Goldenseal (*Hydrastis canadensis*)

Berberine, a compound in this well-used herb, gives goldenseal its ability to soothe the mucous membranes of the digestive, genitourinary, and respiratory tracts when they are inflamed by allergy or infection. Berberine has also been shown to fight *Candida albicans* (yeast) and other fungi, and bacteria such as salmonellae, staphylococci, and streptococci.

Goldenseal is a popular herb, particularly in prepared combinations with echinacea. I suggest goldenseal for treating chronic constipation, conjunctivitis, eczema, and tonsillitis, but only if the severity of the illness or condition warrants it. If you think your child could benefit from goldenseal, consult an herbalist or other medical practitioner. Goldenseal is a potent herb, and a skilled herbal practitioner can help you assess the need for it, help prescribe appropriate dosages, or assist you in finding an alternative.

CAUTIONS: Long-term use of goldenseal can decrease the absorption of vitamin B and reduce intestinal bacteria. Large doses may cause vomiting and diarrhea, slow the pulse, and result in paralysis of the respiratory system. Although topical use is common, strong extracts of goldenseal may cause skin ulcers.

CONTRAINDICATIONS: Goldenseal should not be given to children unless prescribed by a professional (see Additional Cautions, page 58).

Greater celandine (*Chelidonium majus*)

Greater celandine is used in ointments for eczema, hemorrhoids, and wounds. The sap from the fresh plant, applied twice a day, will also heal warts.

CONTRAINDICATIONS: Greater celandine can cause dizziness, dry mouth, and skin irritation.

Helichrysum (*Helichrysum angustifolia*)

As an antibacterial, helichrysum essential oil helps heal bruises, cuts, minor burns, and scrapes, and is an important ingredient in remedies for skin problems, such as abscesses, boils, dermatitis, eczema, psoriasis, and other irritations. It's also used in lotions, mud masks, skin creams, and toners. As an antiviral, it is effective in the treatment of colds and warts. As an antifungal, it fights athlete's foot, fungal infections of the scalp, nail fungus, and ringworm. In a diffuser, it can help respiratory problems.

CONTRAINDICATIONS: Helichrysum is generally considered safe, but some literature suggests young children should not use the herb. The herb may be used in remedies for older children, but only if properly diluted.

Hibiscus (*Hibiscus sabdariffa*)

Hibiscus makes a tart-sweet, red tea that children love. Combined with a little fruit juice, hibiscus can be an ingredient in tasty popsicles. This palatable and potent antioxidant can be used for conditions as varied as digestive conditions (lack of appetite, constipation, gastritis, gastroenteritis, upset stomach), respiratory illnesses (breathing problems, colds and flu, cough, laryngitis, phlegm, sore throat), skin conditions, and urinary problems.

Hops (*Humulus lupulus*)

Hops is known as an ingredient in beer, of course, but in herbal medicine, it's used to promote sleep, relieve pain, and calm a nervous stomach. I tend not to prescribe it too often for children because it is a strong-acting herb. Hops is known to cause long, deep sleep, and I believe that children need to be able to awaken freely. I do recommend hops as an ingredient in "dream pillows" for children. A dream pillow or sachet usually contains equal parts of dried chamomile, hops, and lavender, and is placed near the child's bed to help him sleep.

CONTRAINDICATIONS: Hops is too strong for infants. Babies younger than two years of age should not be given hops under any circumstances (see Additional Cautions, page 58). Children being treated for depression should not be given hops unless advised by a doctor or health-care practitioner. Hops should not be taken with other sedative drugs.

Horehound (*Marrubium vulgare*)

Because of its antiseptic and expectorant properties, horehound is commonly found in cold and cough remedies, such as cough syrups, lozenges, and teas. Horehound is often included in remedies to treat bronchitis, flu, and sinusitis. It also increases perspiration, relieves spasms, stimulates bile flow, and has a calming effect on the heart.

Horseradish (*Armoracia rusticana*)

You may know horseradish only as a spicy condiment, but horseradish has a rich medicinal history. It is an antibacterial, a diaphoretic, and improves circulation, making it one of the herbs to turn to for poultices and herbal blends to relieve arthritic and rheumatic joints, chilblains, chronic rheumatism, muscular aches and pains, and paralytic complaints. Horseradish can help reduce fever, heal urinary tract infections, and improve digestion. It is also known for its ability to break up chest congestion and mucus in the respiratory tract, so it's popular in remedies that treat asthma, bronchitis, colds, coughs (including those that are dry or persistent), emphysema, flu, sinus infections, and whooping cough. Its sharp pungency helps to clear sinuses in one breath. (Expect it to bring tears to your eyes.) If you like to eat horseradish, be sure to add some to your diet if you feel a cough or a cold coming on.

CONTRAINDICATIONS: Children younger than four years of age should not be given horseradish for medicinal purposes.

Ivy (*Glechoma hederacea*)

Ivy has spasmolytic, secretolytic, and mild sedative effects. Remedies containing ivy are used to quell congestion, coughs, and nervous tension headaches. Traditionally, this herb has been used to remove lead from the body by causing it to be secreted in the urine.

Jojoba (*Simmondsia chinensis*)

When whaling was banned, jojoba sprang to importance, replacing whale oil in skin-care and cosmetic products. Jojoba "oil" (it's actually a wax) has a chemical makeup similar to the oil our skin produces naturally. In fact, jojoba is one of the most easily absorbed vegetable oils available. It is used for skin conditions, such as eczema, psoriasis, and rosacea. It is also a common ingredient in massage oils.

Lady's mantle (*Alchemilla vulgaris*)

Lady's mantle is primarily used as an ingredient in remedies for women's health issues, such as, endometriosis, excessive menstrual bleeding, fibroids, painful or irregular periods, and vaginal discharge. As a mouthwash or gargle, it is beneficial for bleeding gums. As a wash or compress, it is used on insect bites, cuts, and scrapes. As tea, it is helpful for diarrhea and gastroenteritis.

Lavender (*Lavandula officinalis*)

It may be the most romantic, aromatic herb, but lavender's calming and antibiotic properties are useful in medicinal, culinary, and cosmetic applications. Used in remedies for anxiety, depression, headache, and nervous exhaustion, lavender also helps promote sleep in children. Keep lavender oil on hand for bruises, cuts, headaches, scrapes, and bedtime foot rubs.

Lemon balm (*Melissa officinalis*)

Lemon balm is great for anxiety, depression, digestive disorders, headache, restlessness and stress. It is also an antiviral. I prescribe lemon balm for cold sores and headaches, and for calming nervous or stressed-out kids (and parents). It has a glorious aroma, and most children like the taste. Because of its high essential oil content, it's best to use the fresh herb, which can increasingly be found in the supermarket produce section near the fresh basil plants.

Licorice (*Glycyrrhiza glabra*)

Licorice is an anti-inflammatory, an antiviral, a demulcent, and an expectorant. It's an ingredient in remedies for coughs, constipation, and ulcerating skin conditions. Used topically, it helps clear up eczema, herpes, insect bites, shingles, and sunburn.

CAUTIONS: The excessive use of licorice can be toxic. Too much licorice may cause edema, elevated blood pressure, headaches, hypertension, lethargy, or shortness of breath. Babies younger than two years of age should not be given licorice under any circumstances (see Additional Cautions, page 58).

Marjoram (*Origanum majorana*)

In a tea or a compress, marjoram helps soothe headaches, the digestive tract, and the stomach. As a compress, it's beneficial for bruises and minor cuts and scrapes, and it's a great addition to liniments. It also helps clear congestion and alleviate asthma.

CONTRAINDICATIONS: Marjoram is contraindicated in kids who are allergic to the mint family (basil, hyssop, lavender, oregano, sage, thyme, and so on).

Marshmallow (*Althaea officinalis*)

Marshmallow is often used for soothing inflamed mucous membranes or any time a soothing remedy is needed. It is also used to treat conditions such as asthma, cough, Crohn's disease, diarrhea, gastritis, gastroesophageal reflux disease, indigestion, peptic ulcer, and ulcerative colitis. As a compress, it is beneficial for minor wounds and skin irritations. As a tea, it can be beneficial for colds, sore throats, and urinary tract inflammations.

Meadowsweet (*Filipendula ulmaria*)

Meadowsweet is an anti-inflammatory and is a good choice for sore muscles and aches and pains. Try it in a soak or compress to relieve joint pain, rheumatism, sprains, and toothache. Its effectiveness in pain relief also extends to headaches, and many people find relief from migraines with remedies that include meadowsweet. The herb also is an astringent that is helpful for diarrhea and bladder infection.

Motherwort (*Leonurus cardiaca*)

Motherwort is the herbal remedy for anxiety, fear, and worry, and it is an excellent heart tonic. Research confirms its ability to calm irregular heartbeat, palpitations, and rapid heartbeat, specifically tachycardia caused by anxiety. It can also be used for all heart conditions associated with anxiety and tension. In children, it's good for new-school or first-day-at-school anxiety.

Mullein (*Verbascum thapsus*)

Another versatile herb, mullein is highly effective in treating spastic coughs and upper and lower respiratory infections. It is often prescribed for earache, catarrhal deafness, and other diseases of the ear, as well as for asthma, bronchitis, ulcerations, and urinary tract inflammation. Mullein is an anodyne, a demulcent, and a diuretic, and it has antispasmodic properties. Infused mullein flower is most commonly used as an ear oil for infections, but it is also commonly prescribed for hemorrhoids, sore throats, and tonsillitis. It's a must-have for the family apothecary.

Mustard (*Brassica alba* and *B. nigra*)

This herb is known for stimulating circulation, so it's great for muscular and skeletal aches and pains, and is often an ingredient in liniments and ointments. It also helps relieve colds and flu. As an infusion or poultice, it helps relieve bronchitis.

CONTRAINDICATIONS: Children under the age of six years should not use this herb medicinally. Pay close attention to the amounts called for in remedies, and do not use more mustard than specified.

Myrrh (*Commiphora myrrha*)

Myrrh is the reddish-brown resin or sap from myrrh trees. Because of its effective antimicrobial properties, it is prescribed for mouth sores, sinusitis, and urinary tract infections.

CONTRAINDICATIONS: Larger doses can irritate the kidneys and cause diarrhea.

Nutmeg (*Myristica fragrans*)

These days, nutmeg is used primarily as a spice in cooking and baking, but it is also included in some medicinal remedies to alleviate colic, diarrhea, gastrointestinal disorders, and vomiting.

CAUTIONS: In large amounts, nutmeg can cause hallucinations and elation, somewhat like marijuana. Large doses can also produce delirium, double vision, stomach pain, and other symptoms of poisoning. It is safe to use in normal amounts for baking and cooking, but it can be dangerous if misused. Eating as few as two nutmegs can cause death.

Oats, milky oats, or oat straw (*Avena sativa*)

Using this herb is as simple as eating oatmeal for breakfast. Oats, generally called by their Latin name, *Avena*, in herbal medicine, are beneficial to the nervous system. It helps to calm and relax the body. Topically, oats can be used in bath water to lessen skin irritation, particularly itching from chicken pox, eczema, hives, and measles. In Europe, oats are used to treat herpes simplex, herpes zoster, and shingles.

Orange flower (*Citrus sinensis*)

Orange essential oil helps clear congestion, so it's beneficial for colds and flu. As a massage oil, it helps alleviate constipation and slow digestion. It is applied topically to brighten the skin. As a diffusion, orange essential oil helps relieve stress and exhaustion, making it a good choice in remedies for bed-wetting. Children may wet the bed due to insecurities, trauma, or an upheaval. This oil promotes relaxation, a feeling of calm, and well-being.

CAUTIONS: Orange essential oil can cause phototoxicity, so do not give it to children before they go out in the sun. Make sure the oil is diluted before applying topically since it can irritate the skin.

Oregano (*Origanum vulgare*)

Another highly versatile herb that can be found in almost every kitchen, oregano is included in scores of herbal remedies. It is high in antioxidants, so it fights free radicals that damage cells. It is an antimicrobial and can fight foodborne pathogens, including *Listeria monocytogenes*. In many parts of the world, oregano is used primarily as a medicine since it helps so many conditions, including colds, flu, fungal infections, parasites, sore throats, stomach and respiratory illnesses, and unrestful sleep. And, applied topically, it is an antiseptic.

CONTRAINDICATIONS: When used topically, oregano must be diluted according to the recipe to prevent contact dermatitis. (This does not apply to oil of oregano, which is a different product.)

Osha root (*Ligusticum porteri*)

Osha has been shown to act against bacteria, viruses, and yeast. It contains compounds that promote immunity and break infection, so it's a good remedy for bronchial and sinus infections, colds, flu, laryngitis, and sore throat when given at the first sign of illness. It's also used in arthritis remedies and for carpal tunnel syndrome.

CONTRAINDICATIONS: Osha is not considered safe for younger children when given internally. Osha root should not be given internally to children unless prescribed by a professional (see Additional Cautions, page 58).

Parsley (*Petroselinum crispum*)

Parsley is more than a garnish on your dinner plate: It's an ingredient in remedies for anemia and constipation. It can also be given as a tea at the onset of a fever.

CONTRAINDICATIONS: Although parsley is regarded as a safe food, it has been shown to cause kidney inflammation when used medicinally.

Passionflower (*Passiflora incarnata*)

Passionflower is often prescribed as a sedative. It relieves anxiety, stress, and related emotional conditions, and it can help with insomnia. Passionflower is an antispasmodic that is effective in compresses, liniments, and poultices for relieving back pain, headache, sore muscles, and neuralgia, including nerve pain such as sciatica and shingles. Passionflower is also prescribed in remedies for diarrhea and dysentery. As a compress, it relieves the pain of hemorrhoids.

CAUTIONS: Passionflower can cause drowsiness and increase the effect of prescription sedatives. Do not administer more than recommended levels, and do not combine with prescription sedatives.

CONTRAINDICATIONS: Children age ten and younger should not be given passionflower.

Patchouli (*Pogostemon cablin*)

Almost everyone is familiar with the scent of patchouli. (People either love it or hate it; it's one of those things.) As a compress, lotion, skin wash, or toner, it is beneficial for athlete's foot, chapped skin, dermatitis, eczema, and oily skin. In a diffuser, it is beneficial for fatigue and stress.

Peppermint (*Mentha piperita*)

Is there a more popular herb than peppermint? Topically, peppermint is used as a tincture or liniment to relieve sore muscles and strains. Internally, it soothes the gastrointestinal tract by relaxing the muscles of the intestinal wall, making it a good remedy for colic, flatulence, gastritis, irritable bowl syndrome, motion sickness, nausea, and stomach and intestinal cramps. In addition, peppermint increases the production of saliva, which increases swallowing and stimulates the appetite and digestion.

Peppermint tea and tincture relieve cold and cough symptoms and bacterial, fungal, respiratory, and viral infections. The oil may be mixed with steamy water and inhaled to soothe nasal passages that are irritated by allergies or a sinus infection. (See Inhalation Therapy, page 74.)

Peppermint is often beneficial for headaches that are associated with digestive problems. It is also included in remedies for nervous tension and anxiety. Because it is gentle, I like to suggest a simple peppermint tea for most children's conditions. Peppermint can also be used as an extract, infused oil, salve, or tincture.

CONTRAINDICATIONS: Due to its choleretic activity, peppermint should not be used by anyone with gallstones.

Periwinkle (*Vinca major*)

Periwinkle is a great astringent that is useful both internally and externally. Generally, it is prescribed for conditions involving the urinary tract. As a gargle, it helps heal bleeding gums, mouth ulcers, and sore throats. As a compress, periwinkle kills the pain of wasp and bee stings, relieves eye inflammation, and stops bleeding.

CAUTIONS: Improper use of periwinkle can thin the blood and cause other problems; follow directions carefully when giving periwinkle internally. If in doubt, use only externally.

Pine (*Pinus sylvestris*)

Pine is used in medications all over the world, but unfortunately it's not as popular in the United States as it once was. I think American herbalists should take a closer look at pine. The tea is used topically to treat eczema and internally for colds, flu, and other bronchial complaints. Pine is also used in inhalation therapy to clear the sinuses.

Plantain (*Plantago major*)

Plantain has strongly astringent and soothing properties, and helps to reduce the pain of insect bites, stings, and wounds. It also helps stop bleeding. Fortunately, it's one of the most widespread herbs on the planet, so it's easy to find.

Plantain is used in poultices and applied topically for bites, boils, cuts, scrapes, and stings. In a salve, it can be used anytime a child gets a bump or a scrape. Plantain can also be taken internally as an infusion for burning diarrhea, intestinal upsets, and sore throat.

Purple loosestrife (*Lythrum salicaria*)

Because of its astringent properties, purple loosestrife is traditionally used in treating dysentery and diarrhea. It's also helpful as an eye rinse or in a compress for conjunctivitis (pink eye).

Although the herb is plentiful in the wild—it's a noxious weed, so don't plant it unless you can restrain it—purple loosestrife products aren't readily available. You may have to hunt for them.

CONTRAINDICATIONS: Purple loosestrife is generally considered safe, although little is mentioned in the literature.

Ravensara (*Ravensara aromatica*)

Ravensara essential oil has strong antiviral properties and is essential for treating colds and flu. In a diffuser or in steam inhalation therapy, the essential oil helps heal sinus infections and provides relief for coughs and colds. As a massage preparation, it relaxes muscles and relieves tension and muscle strains. Ravensara also makes a good cleanser to help prevent flu outbreaks in the family. To make the cleanser, simply combine thirty to sixty drops of ravensara essential oil with eight ounces of water in a spray bottle.

Red clover (*Trifolium pratense*)

Red clover is a gorgeous flower, and my children used to love to pick it when they were toddlers. (My youngest used to ask for the flowers in salads.)

Red clover purifies and detoxifies the blood. It is a mild antispasmodic, anti-inflammatory, expectorant, and sedative. It is very effective in bedtime teas and cough syrups. Parents tell me it substantially calms the "whoop" of whooping cough.

Eczema, psoriasis, and other skin issues can all benefit from red clover compresses, infused oil, tea, and washes. As a tea or tincture, red clover eases headaches, hormonal imbalances, migraines, and PMS. In addition, it relieves fibromyalgia, gastrointestinal disorders, and irritable bowel syndrome.

CONTRAINDICATIONS: Red clover is generally considered safe for children when used for short and reasonable periods of time.

Red raspberry leaf (*Rubus idaeus*)

Red raspberry leaf acts as an astringent, meaning it is helpful in reducing secretions and discharges. It often is used in remedies for anemia, canker sores, colic, diarrhea, and gastrointestinal upset. Raspberry leaf tea is also an anti-inflammatory and can be used as a gargle for sore throats.

Red sage

See Sage, page 51.

Rose hips/rose (*Rosa rugosa* or *R. canina*)

This is one of my favorite herbs because it tastes great and is a nutritional powerhouse, helping to build up the body during times of illness and weakness. Rose hips contain carotenoids, flavonoids, pectins, and vitamins C and E. It has a gentle laxative effect, which can assist with constipation. Often, it is added to other remedies simply for its nutritional value and delicious flavor.

Rose petals (*Rosa canina*)

Rose petals have powerful antibacterial, anti-inflammatory, and antioxidant actions. Rose petal water can be used as an eyewash and mouthwash, and the petals can be blended into a face mask for general skin cleansing.

CONTRAINDICATIONS: Rose petals are generally considered safe but should not be given to children with rose allergies.

Rosemary (*Rosmarinus officinalis*)

Rosemary is a nervous system stimulant but has a calming effect on digestion. It's prescribed for depression, headaches, and muscular pain.

Rosemary tincture can be used for stomach and nervous system issues. It can also be used as a salve, an ointment, and a massage oil for aches and pains, circulation issues, and sore tendons and ligaments. Rosemary salve on your temples will ease a headache; on your cheeks, it will improve a sinus condition; and on your neck, it will relieve tension.

CAUTIONS: Used topically, rosemary may cause skin irritation.

CONTRAINDICATIONS: Although generally considered safe, rosemary can be dangerous in extremely large doses. Children with epilepsy, diverticulosis, chronic ulcers, colitis, or high blood pressure should not be given rosemary internally for medicinal purposes.

Rosewood (Aniba rosaeodora)

Rosewood is popularly used in the treatment of dry, oily, and sensitive skin. It also is beneficial for colds, flu, headaches, and stress when used in the bath, in a diffuser, or in steam inhalation therapy.

Rue (Ruta graveolens)

Rue has been used for centuries for cough and colic. Because its antispasmodic capabilities relax smooth muscles, the herb is helpful in relieving tension in the digestive tract. Rue also increases circulation to the extremities, helps lower elevated blood pressure, and can relieve tension headaches and anxiety issues.

CONTRAINDICATIONS: Rue should not be given to children unless prescribed by a professional (see Additional Cautions, page 58).

Sage/red sage (Salvia officinalis)

In Latin, the word "sage" means wisdom and good taste. I love sage for so many remedies, especially for children, because it is easy to find fresh, it is inexpensive, and its anti-inflammatory and antioxidant properties make it gentle and powerful at the same time.

Sage-based remedies are effective for laryngitis, mouth inflammation, sore or bleeding gums, sore throats, tonsillitis, and as a compress for wounds. Sage is also used in remedies for headaches, and for diarrhea in babies.

Skullcap (Scutellaria lateriflora)

Skullcap is a safe and effective nerve tonic, prescribed for hyperactivity, mental and anxiety disorders (especially those linked to school pressures), shaking, and tremors. (For emotional problems, skullcap can be used in small dosages over a period of time.) Skullcap is also an ingredient in remedies for arthritis and headache, especially headaches behind the eye. Used topically and internally, it dulls the sting of insect bites and also is given for insomnia.

CAUTIONS: An overdose can cause confusion, giddiness, stupor, and twitching.

CONTRAINDICATIONS: Do not combine skullcap with blood thinners, sedatives, or sleeping pills.

Sea holly (Eryngium maritimum)

This herb is a powerful diuretic that is often used in cases of urinary tract infection and gravel in the urinary system. The candied root is used as a remedy for cough. Sea holly is also beneficial for asthma, general bladder issues, and nervous dispositions.

Slippery elm (Ulmus rubra)

Slippery elm is a mucilaginous herb, which means it is a soothing demulcent. Useful in lubricating inflamed mucous linings, it quiets intestinal irritation and the nervous system. It's prescribed for diarrhea, gastric ulcers, gastritis, sore throat, and as an overall nutritious gruel when a child feels ill.

The most widely used part of the plant is the bark, which is used as a decoction. (In order for it to mix completely, it should be tempered first by adding one part powdered bark to eight parts water.)

Spearmint leaf (Mentha spicata)

Spearmint reduces muscle spasms in the stomach, so it has been used traditionally to relieve gas, indigestion, and nausea. It is high in vitamins A and C. Because of its pronounced flavor, it is often added to herbal remedies to mask bad-tasting ingredients.

St. John's wort (Hypericum perforatum)

St. John's wort is the infused oil of choice for many infant-care products because of its powerful anti-inflammatory, astringent, nervine, and vulnerary capabilities. The infused oil feels like sunshine when applied to the skin and can be used topically for bruises, mild burns, and sores. I've also used it for my children's skin problems, such as diaper rash or dry or irritated skin, and when they have sore backs or necks. It's an herb with truly amazing capabilities.

Before St. John's wort became popular as an antidepressant, it was the go-to herb for many other conditions, including nerve pain, sciatica, sunburn, and varicose veins. Its salve or oil is a remedy for all types of skin problems, including severe eczema, psoriasis, and teething rash. It can be used topically, in infused oil form or as a tincture, to treat a child's sore muscles after physical activity and for any postaccident or postsurgical bruising. Many of my clients have used it on surgical scars when they start hurting or itching, and it has offered them significant relief.

As a tea, St. John's wort quiets and relaxes the mind. It is also taken internally for anxiety, bed-wetting, depression, nervous disposition, and traumatic shock.

CAUTIONS: St. John's wort can cause photosensitivity in some children, so make sure children who are taking it use sunblock and wear sun hats when they go out in the sun.

CONTRAINDICATIONS: If your child is taking prescription antidepressants, be sure to check with your doctor before using St. John's wort. It should not be used for severe depression, and it should not be used with monoamine oxidase (MAO) inhibitors.

Stinging nettle (Urtica dioica)

Stinging nettle, or just "nettle," has traditionally been used to strengthen and support the whole body. It can be eaten as a food or used medicinally as a tea, tincture, extract, or in capsule form. Rich in chlorophyll, calcium, and iron, nettle is high in protein, ascorbic acid, magnesium, and vitamin K. These nutrients work together to promote healthy bones, joints, and skin and encourage a healthy immune and respiratory system. Stinging nettle can be used for diarrhea, eczema, hay fever, and sore joints. Because this herb is so versatile, it can be a good tonic remedy to "hide" in foods to boost nutrition. I add it to casseroles, pasta, and risotto.

CONTRAINDICATIONS: Nettle has been shown to enhance the effect of the nonsteroidal anti-inflammatory drug diclofenac. Consult a doctor before administering a nettle remedy if your child is taking diclofenac. Nettle also is contraindicated in cases of fluid retention from decreased renal function and reduced cardiac function.

Sundew (*Drosera rotundifolia*)

Well-known as a carnivorous plant with a penchant for insects, sundew also has antispasmodic, antitussive, demulcent, and expectorant properties that make it a good remedy for cough. Sundew treats asthma and chronic bronchitis, bronchial and dry cough, whooping cough, and other types of dry, persistent coughs.

CONTRAINDICATIONS: Sundew may cause allergic reactions in some children but is generally regarded as safe.

Tea tree (*Melaleuca alternifolia*)

Tea tree oil is an essential oil extracted from the melaleuca tree. It is always used as an external remedy. These days, this wildly popular herb is found in everything from athlete's foot preparations to toothpaste. Its antibiotic properties also help treat candida, chicken pox, colds, cold sores, cuts, dandruff, flu, insect bites, ringworm, sinusitis, and even flea infestations. Tea tree essential oil can be added to balms, liniments, lotions, and salves.

Tea tree essential oil has been found to be antiseptic and antifungal, and it is a favorite in my house for cleaning and deodorizing. I add a few drops to laundry when one of my family members is sick. When I use it to clean surfaces that transmit germs, such as door knobs, faucets, and toilet handles, I find that illness is wiped out much faster. I passed this tip on to a student who runs a daycare center, and she said that it seemed to cut down on illness there as well.

CAUTIONS: Tea tree essential oil should not be used for children age six and younger unless it is diluted. (Refer to the individual remedy recipes and information about essential oils in chapter 5, page 120.) Otherwise, it is generally regarded as safe.

CONTRAINDICATIONS: As with any essential oil, tea tree essential oil should not be taken internally. Do not apply to mucous membranes or put inside children's ears without proper dilution.

Thuja (*Thuja occidentalis*)

Thuja is used in foot washes and compresses as an antifungal, and in cough syrups and teas as an expectorant. As an infused oil, it can be used for the topical treatment of warts and herpes cold sores.

CAUTIONS: Thuja can be toxic if the recommended dosage is exceeded; follow dosage instructions carefully. Thuja is not for long-term use.

CONTRAINDICATIONS: Children with liver or kidney impairment should not be given thuja. Thuja should not be given to children unless prescribed by a professional (see Additional Cautions, page 58).

Thyme (*Thymus vulgaris*)

Although indigenous to the Mediterranean, thyme is abundant all over North America and Europe. This wonderful herb is a powerful antimicrobial, antiseptic, antispasmodic, astringent, and expectorant, and it has been used in the treatment of whooping cough for hundreds of years. The German Commission E approved its use for whooping cough based on the herb's bronchial spasmolytic, expectorant, and antibacterial capabilities. (In Germany, only herbs with Commission E approval are available legally.)

In addition to its use in the treatment of whooping cough, and for coughs and colds in general, thyme is also included in remedies for colic, headache, neuralgia, and sluggish digestion. Because it is also an astringent, it is helpful in the treatment of bed-wetting and diarrhea.

CAUTIONS: Thyme's taste can be a little strong for children; however, adding a drop of agave nectar or honey can help the medicinal tea go down.

CONTRAINDICATIONS: Thyme essential oil is highly toxic when ingested internally—even one milliliter can cause poisoning. Habitual use of thyme can cause intestinal irritation. Do not use thyme in remedies for children with liver or kidney disease.

Usnea (*Usnea barbata*)

Usnea is a lichen, that is, an alga and a fungus, that has a long history of use by North American herbalists, mostly as an alternative for people who do not respond to the popular herb echinacea. Usnea has been shown to block bacteria metabolism, making it an effective antibiotic, and it is used very successfully in the treatment of bronchitis, colds, flu, pneumonia, respiratory and urinary infections, sinus infections, strep and staph infections, and tuberculosis. Usnea is also used to treat urogenital problems, such as bacterial vaginosis and vaginal yeast infections.

Valerian (*Valeriana officinalis*)

Valerian is popularly known as a sleep-inducing herb. In addition, it is often used in remedies for headache, especially for tension headaches and migraines. It is also added to cough remedies to calm spasmodic coughing and relieve muscle tension in the chest. Valerian can also be found in many PMS remedies. It helps calm cramps and relieve painful menstruation (dysmenorrhea).

CAUTIONS: Studies have suggested that valerian is generally regarded as safe to use for short periods of time, four to six weeks, for example. Valerian can have mild side effects, such as dizziness, headaches, tiredness, and upset stomach, the morning after its use.

CONTRAINDICATIONS: Children younger than twelve years of age should not be given valerian internally. Babies younger than two years of age should not be given valerian under any circumstance. (See Additional Cautions, page 58.)

White oak bark (*Quercus robur*)

An astringent, white oak bark is used to tighten tissues and blood vessels, making it an ingredient in remedies for conditions as diverse as diarrhea, gum disease, hemorrhoids, and varicose veins. As an anti-inflammatory, it is prescribed for inflammations and irritations caused by poor digestion, skin problems, strep throat, and ulcers. It can also be beneficial for bites, bleeding, and dental problems.

CONTRAINDICATIONS: Do not use white oak bark for more than two days at a time. If necessary, use it for two days, then skip a day before using it for two more days, then skip a day, and so on. Do not use externally on skin with burns, cuts, or scrapes. Children with heart disease, wet eczema, or any illness that includes fever should not bathe in white oak bark.

Wild cherry bark (*Prunus serotina*)

At one time, wild cherry bark was an ingredient in almost every over-the-counter cough syrup, and no wonder. It is an antitussive, an antispasmodic, an astringent, an expectorant, and a nervine. Wild cherry bark is often included in remedies for especially irritating coughs and is used to treat bronchitis, colds, and whooping cough. It helps that kids love the flavor.

Wild cherry bark has other uses in herbal medicine as well. The tea, prepared as a decoction and cooled, is used in a compress to soothe eye inflammations. In addition, it is helpful for treating nervous debility and chronic weak digestion.

CAUTIONS: Although the leaves are considered poisonous, wild cherry bark is generally regarded as safe; use only the bark. With excessive use, wild cherry bark can cause drowsiness and other issues.

Wild indigo (*Baptisia tinctoria*)

Wild indigo, an effective antiseptic, is used to clean wounds and as a treatment for ear, nose, throat, and sinus infections. Wild indigo is great for preventing and treating the flu.

CAUTIONS: Large doses can cause diarrhea, paralysis of the respiratory system, and vomiting and other gastrointestinal issues; follow usage instructions carefully.

CONTRAINDICATIONS: Children with autoimmune disorders should not be given wild indigo.

Wild yam (*Dioscorea villosa*)

Wild yam is mostly known for its ability to normalize hormonal imbalances, but it is also used for many other types of conditions, including stomach cramps and muscle aches and pains.

Witch hazel leaf (*Hamamelis virginiana*)

Witch hazel is an astringent and an excellent choice for most skin-care problems. It has been used for years as an aftershave lotion and for treating cracked or blistered skin, eczema, hemorrhoids, insect bites, poison ivy, psoriasis, and varicose veins. It can be found in many over-the-counter products.

Witch hazel is mainly used externally on bruises, sores, and swelling. It can be used as a compress, liniment, tea, tincture, and wash.

CAUTIONS: Do not take witch hazel internally.

Yarrow *(Achillea millefolium)*

Yarrow is a wound-healing herb. I once placed crushed fresh yarrow on a knee gash I got while hiking and saw an immediate end to the bleeding. Yarrow is anti-inflammatory, antispasmodic, astringent, diuretic, and reduces fever. It is helpful in remedies for internal bleeding and bruising and swelling, especially in the ankles. (It is easy to wrap the plant around a wrist or ankle.)

CONTRAINDICATIONS: Yarrow should be used with caution in children who are allergic to ragweed.

Yellow dock root *(Rumex crispus)*

Yellow dock decoction and tincture are helpful for digestive problems, such as constipation and indigestion, and for skin disorders, such as eczema and psoriasis. It is also a mild laxative and helps heal boils and fungal infections.

CAUTIONS: Yellow dock root and other plants of the Polygonaceae family contain oxalates in their leaves and should not be eaten by anyone with kidney stones.

ADDITIONAL CAUTIONS

Many of the following herbs are not mentioned in this chapter because they should not be used to treat babies or children. Of the herbs that were mentioned, some should be used only when prescribed by a professional.

Herbs That Should Not Be Given to Babies

Babies younger than two years of age should *not* be given the following herbs *under any circumstances*:

Cayenne *(Capsicum frutescens)*: This herb is too spicy and hot for infants.

Echinacea (*Echinacea purpurea*): Echinacea's safety has not been evaluated in babies.

Ephedra or ma huang (*Ephedra sinensis*): In the United States, it has been illegal to sell supplements containing the drug ephedrine since 2004. The sale of the herb ephedra is regulated in the United States, although the drug and the herb are technically different. Ephedrine is a constituent of the herb, not the whole herb itself. Ephedra can cause nervousness and anxiety in children.

Hops (*Humulus lupulus*): Hops' ability to induce sleep is too strong for infants.

Licorice (*Glycyrrhiza glabra*): Licorice can have negative effects on the liver with long-term use, which is dangerous for infants.

Valerian (*Valeriana officinalis*): Valerian is a sleep-inducing herb. Although generally regarded as safe, valerian should not be given to children younger than four years of age because it is essential for children to learn their own sleep patterns. Because valerian works so well, there is the danger of overuse.

Herbs That Should Not Be Given to Babies or Children

Children younger than twelve should *not* be given the following herbs *internally*:

Arnica (*Arnica montana*): Use the homeopathic form only; the straight herb is poisonous.

Buckthorn (*Rhamnus cathartica*): Buckthorn is a strong laxative that can cause diarrhea and deplete potassium levels.

Cascara sagrada (*Rhamnus purshiana*) **and senna** (*Cassia angustifolia* and *C. senna*): These herbs are strong laxatives and can cause diarrhea, intestinal cramps, and stomach cramps. With proper dosing, the herbs may be appropriate for adults, but not for infants and children.

Comfrey (*Symphytum officinale*): Both British and U.S. regulatory bodies have issued warnings about comfrey and the toxicity of compounds called *pyrrolizidine alkaloids*, which may cause liver damage when the herb is used internally. Only the leaf form is safe for internal use, but it should only be given to children over ten years of age. However, topical use of comfrey in creams, oils, ointments, poultices, and tinctures is generally regarded to be safe.

Ephedra or ma huang: See Herbs That Should Not Be Given to Babies, page 59.

Pennyroyal (*Mentha pulegium* or *Hedeoma pulegioides*): Pennyroyal is no longer considered safe for use in children. It can be toxic to the nerves and liver.

Poke root (*Phytolacca decandra*): Poke should never be given to childen. An overdose can cause nausea, vomiting, oral irritation, cramps, slowed respiration, drowsiness, tingling sensations throughout the body, overall weakness, profuse sweating, convulsions, and reduced blood pressure and pulse. Used topically, it can cause contact dermatitis and irritation. If the consumption of poke is greater than one-half ounce of the berries or root, or ten berries in an infant, coma and death by respiratory paralysis could occur.

Southernwood (*Artemisia abrotanum*): Southernwood can cause insomnia, nausea, and vertigo and should not be used by children or anyone taking phenobarbital.

Valerian: See Herbs That Should Not Be Given to Babies, page 59.

Wormwood (*Artemisia absinthium*): Wormwood is too strong for children and also is a uterine stimulant.

Herbs that Should Only Be Prescribed by a Professional

Babies and children should use the following herbs only when they are administered by an experienced herbalist or a medical practitioner:

Barberry (*Berberis vulgaris*): Burning, itching, and redness have been documented following topical applications of remedies containing barberry. Reactions include symptoms of poisoning, such as daze, diarrhea, lethargy, nephritis, stupor, and vomiting.

Beth root (*Trillium erectum*): Beth root has not yet been observed in clinical situations, but it may irritate membranes and have cardiac effects.

Calendula (*Calendula officinalis*): Infants and small children should not be given calendula internally because it can potentially cause allergic reactions and sensitization.

Cotton root (*Gossypium herbaceum*): This herb has a tendency to cause irritation and inflammation of the urogenital tract, and there is some indication that it can cause sterility in males.

Feverfew (*Chrysanthemum parthenium*): This herb should not be given to children younger than two years of age. Headaches, mouth ulcers, and stomach issues have been reported with improper use. Feverfew can cause allergic reactions in children with allergies to this plant family.

Goldenseal (*Hydrastis canadensis*): Taken internally, goldenseal can cause intestinal problems. A compound in goldenseal called berberine may displace bilirubin in babies, which could be a serious problem. Very large doses of the herb could induce anxiety, depression, nausea, paralysis, or seizures in children. These reactions, however, are rare.

Juniper (*Juniperus communis*): Epidermal reactions can occur with juniper, as can allergic reactions in children who are allergic to pollen.

Male fern (*Dryopteris felix-mas*): Some documented adverse reactions include headache and cardiac and respiratory failure. Male fern is considered potentially toxic, and it should be used with care.

Mistletoe (*Viscum album*): Poison control centers report toxicity of the whole plant, but mistletoe berries are especially poisonous. Reactions can include inflammation, itching, and redness. Some systemic reactions include mild fever or flu-like symptoms. Anaphylaxis has been reported.

Mugwort (*Artemisia vulgaris*): The FDA classifies mugwort as unsafe because of its potential degenerative effect on nerves. Some documented reactions have included convulsions, dermatitis, and renal failure.

Osha root (*Ligusticum porteri*): Osha is not considered safe for use in children younger than eight years of age. Some products on the market allow for dosing at younger ages, but these are specially formulated for children. Large dosages can cause stomach irritation. This plant can be confused with poisonous hemlock, so it must be positively identified before using.

Rue (*Ruta graveolens*): Rue has the potential for interactions with drugs that thin the blood. Overdose may cause gastrointestinal irritation, vomiting, renal irritation, liver degeneration, prostration, and death. As a topical application, it can irritate a child's skin and cause blistering, burning, and redness. Internal use of this herb should only be undertaken with the guidance of a trained health-care professional.

Spikenard (*Aralia racemosa*): Problems have occurred with large dosages of spikenard, but not much is known about whether it can be used in smaller dosages.

Tansy (*Tanacetum vulgare*): Tansy can cause irritation and upset.

Thuja (*Thuja occidentalis*): Thuja is toxic if used for long periods and can cause kidney problems. It contains a compound called thujone that is not safe for children.

Remedies for Common Childhood Illnesses

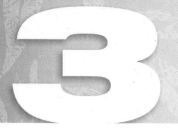

I n spite of all your preventive efforts, kids will get sick. A strong immune system is essential for preventing disease and helping your child fight off illness quickly and dependably. You can help your child build immunity with nutrition. Feed your child a diet abundant in whole grains, legumes, fruit, and vegetables (the more dark, leafy greens and orange and yellow vegetables, the better). It's important to serve foods that are rich in vitamin C and zinc. And always serve water, preferably filtered.

Make sure your kids are physically active year-round, preferably outdoors. Sunshine is the best source of vitamin D. Cow's milk contains small amounts of vitamin D. Because vitamin D is fat-soluble, the fat in whole milk helps it to be metabolized by the body.

Make sure your child gets enough rest. Kids age ten and younger should get ten hours of sleep per night; older children should sleep eight to ten hours. Add an additional hour in winter, a time of regeneration and rest. When children are out in harsh weather, play in the cold or snow, and go to school in the dark and cold, they can become chronically underrested.

Following are descriptions of common childhood illnesses, with suggestions for over-the-counter and homemade herbal remedies for each. Remember, the suggestions in this book should not be a substitute for professional medical advice.

Dosage Guidelines

For young children, always start with the "less is more" approach. In herbal medicine, you may find a tiny dose is all that's needed. To establish the correct dose for your child, take into consideration the ailment, your child's size, the adult dosage, and the form and power of the herb you intend to use. The following guidelines can help:

For extracts and tinctures, start with a dosage of one drop per year of age. For little ones age two and under, always consult your doctor, herbalist, or health-care practitioner about a safe dosage. In general, I tend to give less than one drop to babies age one and under.

For tinctures, follow Young's rule or Clark's rule. Young's rule divides the child's age by twelve *plus* the number equal to the child's age. For example, the dosage for a four-year-old child would be determined by this formula:

$4 \div (12 + 4)$ or 16 = $^4\!/_{16}$ or ¼ of the adult dose

Clark's rule divides the child's weight by 150, so the dosage for a forty-pound child would be determined by this formula:

$40 \div 150$ or $^{40}\!/_{150}$ = 0.27 or about ¼ of the adult dose

For infusions and decoctions, if an adult dose equals one cup, two to three times a day, the following dosages apply to children:

- For children two to four years of age: 2 tablespoons.
- For children five to seven years of age: ¼ cup.
- For children eight to eleven years of age: ½ cup.
- For children twelve years of age and older: ½ to 1 cup.

BED-WETTING

It is normal for toddlers and young children to urinate in their sleep at night. After age five or six, however, bed-wetting, or enuresis, may indicate a slow maturing of the urinary tract (about ten percent of children still wet the bed at age six). Kids usually grow out of this. However, if bed-wetting persists, it could be a symptom of other problems, and you should consult a doctor or health-care practitioner. In the meantime, it is important to remain patient, loving, and accepting.

An Herbal First-Aid Kit

The following herbal products and remedies are good to have on hand for basic first aid:

- aloe vera for burns
- arnica products for sore muscles and bruises
- black tea bags for pain and swelling from insect stings
- ginger candy, capsules, and drinks for nausea, motion sickness, and stomach upsets
- lavender essential oil for burns, cuts, headaches, scrapes, and stress
- peppermint tincture for headaches, insect bites and stings, itching, stomach-aches, and toothaches
- slippery elm capsules or pastilles for diarrhea, food poisoning, and stomach upsets
- tea tree essential oil for burns, cold sores, fungus, and infections
- yarrow to stop bleeding
- an astringent that contains horsetail, rose, St. John's wort, witch hazel, yarrow, and/or yellow dock to treat diarrhea
- a salve that contains calendula, chamomile, chaparral, echinacea, garlic, goldenseal, myrrh, osha, and/or usnea to treat infections
- a salve that contains chickweed, comfrey, marshmallow, plaintain, slippery elm, and/or mullein to treat rashes

To encourage a dry night, withhold liquids three to four hours before your child's bedtime, and take your child to the bathroom just before tucking him in. Children mostly wet the bed when lying on their backs, so suggest that your child sleep in another position.

St. John's wort is helpful for dealing with anxiety and stress, and can also check urination. (Antidepressants are sometimes prescribed to children for this problem because they reduce the amount of urine.) To make St. John's wort tea, pour one cup of boiling water over one teaspoon of dried St. John's wort. Steep the tea at least thirty minutes. Add a little honey to taste (if your child is older than two years of age). Or, try Tea Blend Two (page 135). Give your child two to three cups during the day or at dinner time. Alternatively, give your child five to ten drops of St. John's wort tincture just before bedtime.

Bites and Stings

Bug bites and stings are commonplace during childhood. If children go outside to play, they're going to be subject to them.

I have seen kids with almost every type of bug bite and sting imaginable. Poultices, essential oil blends, and teas for compresses can ease the itch, sting, and swelling. To make sure you're using the most helpful remedy, try to identify the bug or insect. The information in table 1 (below) can help.

Call your child's doctor immediately if

- the bite area blackens; is red, hot, and painful to the touch; oozes pus; or exhibits dead tissue or red streaks;

- your child feels sick or weak, feels achy all over, or is short of breath;

- your child has a fever, headache, or stiff or aching joints or neck;

- your child has a rash near the bite site or anywhere else on the body (other than redness caused by scratching).

When buying prepared bite and sting remedies, look for products that contain one or a combination of the following herbs: aloe vera, calendula, tea tree or lavender oils, and witch hazel. Also look for products that contain plantain, which has strong astringent and

TABLE 1. Bites and stings

TYPE OF BITE	PROBABLE SOURCE OF BITE
Painful	Ant, fly, or spider
Not painful	Spider, mosquito, flea, chigger, or bedbug
Single bite	Mosquito, ant, chigger, or bedbug
Two bites	Spider or tick
Raised, not flat	Spider, ant, flea, or chigger
Flat, not raised, and itchy	Mosquito or fly
Flat, not raised or itchy	Bedbug
Forms a blister	Spider
Does not form a blister	Mosquito, flea, or chigger

soothing properties and helps to reduce the pain of bites, stings, and wounds. It also helps to stop bleeding.

You can also try these simple remedies: Use a cotton swab to dab lavender or tea tree essential oils on the affected area. Soak a bag of black tea, calendula tea, chamomile, green tea, or lemon balm, and apply it directly to the bite. Prepare and apply a compress of black tea, lavender tea, or witch hazel. Or, try St. John's Wort Salve (page 164).

To treat most bites or stings of any type, mix one drop of the essential oil of bergamot, chamomile, lavender, lemon, melissa, or tea tree with one-half teaspoon of water or oil. Apply this to the bite every day. The chamomile version is especially good for bee stings. For mosquito or other insect bites that don't require much attention, a simple dab of essential oil of lavender or tea tree provides relief. Chamomile and lavender essential oils reduce swelling, itching, and inflammation. When used in combination with tinctures of echinacea and plantain, they often prevent an allergic response to bites and stings. (If an allergic reaction does occur, give one-half teaspoon of echinacea tincture internally.)

For a good, quick remedy for gnat bites, mix one teaspoon of apple cider vinegar with two drops of thyme essential oil and one drop of lavender essential oil. Apply this mixture to bites two or three times a day as needed for children older than three years of age. Or, try Insect Bite Gel (page 163), Cootie Oil (page 162), First-Aid Remedy (page 161), or Clay Poultice (page 162).

For a safe, natural bug repellent, try Insect-Aside Bug Repellent (page 163). Or, add two drops lavender essential oil and two drops thyme essential oil to one teaspoon carrier oil (apricot kernel oil or olive oil). Apply directly on the skin to repel bugs and on existing bites to stop itching.

BRUISES

Bruises are of three distinct types: subcutaneous (beneath the skin), intramuscular (inside the underlying muscle), and periosteal (on the outer layer of the bone), which is the most severe and painful type. Bruises can last for a few days to a few months.

Call your child's doctor or health-care practitioner if he is bruising without injuring himself, if there are signs of infection, or if he complains of pain. Never attempt to "drain" a bruise with a needle.

To help heal your child's bruises, use herbal and homeopathic products, such as gels, infused oils, ointments, sprays, and tablets, that contain arnica or lavender. Arnica is renowned for its ability to heal bruising because it stimulates the peripheral blood supply. For small bruises and other minor boo-boos, try First-Aid Remedy (page 161), Plantain-Arnica Compress (page 136), or Plantain Salve (page 174).

Caution: As discussed in chapter 2, never use arnica oil on broken skin. Also, pure arnica essential oil can be toxic. Instead, use infused oil or homeopathic arnica products.

BURNS

In a first-degree burn, minimal tissue damage has occurred and only the outer layer of the skin, or epidermis, has been affected, usually resulting in pain, redness, and swelling. (Serious burns or burns that cover an area larger than your palm should be looked at by a doctor right away.) First-degree burns are extremely sensitive to the touch, and the skin will blanch when light pressure is applied. They require immediate attention. The first step is to run cold water over the affected area to cool the skin and limit the burn. Gently pat the burn dry. After the burn has completely cooled—but *only* after it has cooled—you can apply a topical remedy.

The gel from the aloe vera plant is well-known for its ability to heal burns, often without blisters. Aloe is a demulcent and a vulnerary. In 1973, a study published in the *International Journal of Dermatology* showed that aloe vera has dramatic wound-healing capabilities. Subsequent studies have shown similar results. Aloe vera gel is available in tubes and bottles in almost any drugstore or supermarket. Look for pure aloe vera gel, not lotion. You can also keep a live aloe vera plant in the house. Just cut or break off a leaf or part of a leaf, split it open, and smear the gel onto the burn.

Lavender essential oil also soothes skin and heals burns. It has been used to treat burns for decades and is now used as an adjunct therapy in hospitals. Put a few drops of the oil on a cloth dampened in cold water, and apply it to the burn. You can also prepare a compress using a strong tea made with St. John's wort, and apply it to the burn.

Simple remedies for burns include applying vitamin E oil, comfrey leaf salve, infused oil of St. John's wort, or a thick coating of raw honey. Or, try First-Aid Remedy (page 161), Soothing Salve (page 175), and St. John's Wort Salve (page 164).

CARSICKNESS

Carsickness, also called motion sickness, can upset or even prevent family journeys. Although children age two and younger are rarely affected by it, older kids can suffer from the dizziness, headache, nausea, and vomiting brought on by movement.

Motion sickness occurs when the brain can't rectify contradictory messages from the senses (namely, balance, sight, and touch) that provide information about the body's position. It is triggered when the body is in motion, particularly motion that is rocking and irregular, which can happen in any moving vehicle, including carnival rides.

Prevention is essential. Before and during a trip, your child can avoid motion sickness by eating lightly and passing on heavy foods, junk foods, and foods with strong flavors and aromas. On short plane trips, especially on small planes, he probably shouldn't eat or drink at all. It is best for the child to sit where motion is felt least, such as in the front seat of the car (if he is old enough), the upper deck of a boat, or over the wings of an airplane. He should also sit where there is plenty of fresh air or ventilation, such as near an open car window or on the boat deck. Another way to avoid motion sickness is to face forward. Riding backward confuses the senses. In addition, a child who is prone to motion sickness should not read or look at books in a moving vehicle.

Ginger is an excellent remedy to use just before or during a trip. Give your child products that contain real ginger, not artificial ginger flavoring, such as ginger candies, crystallized ginger, or natural ginger ale. As an alternative, try Motion Sickness Blend (page 168) just before leaving. Cool some of the tea and carry it with you so your child can sip as much as he wants if he begins to feel nauseated. In addition, always carry a few whole-grain crackers in the car just in case.

Motion sickness drugs, including over-the-counter drugs, can have serious side effects in children. They should never be given except under a doctor's supervision.

CHICKEN POX

Chicken pox, caused by the *Varicella zoster* virus, is one of those highly contagious childhood diseases that almost all healthy children recover from; mild cases only require that you treat the symptoms. Most kids with chicken pox will have sores on their the trunk, arms, and legs; headache; moderate fever; loss of appetite; and general malaise. Infants often do not have many of these symptoms. In adults, chicken pox is dangerous and can be fatal.

Two to three days after the symptoms appear, the child will break out with a rash of groups of small, flat, and itchy red spots, usually on the trunk and face, that spread to the arms and legs. The spots become raised with blisters and then crust over. Call your doctor or health-care practitioner if the sores become infected or appear inside the ear, on the eyelids, close to the eyes, or on the end of the penis, making urination difficult.

Mild cases of chicken pox can be treated by easing the itching and keeping your child comfortable. Also, keep your child clean and wash her hands frequently to prevent bacterial infection of the skin. Try either of the skin washes on page 137. If your child has sores in her mouth, keep her hydrated with nonacidic juices, such as apple or pear. Frozen juice bars are soothing. Miso soup is nutritious and healing, so it's a good choice if your child is hungry but her mouth hurts too much to chew.

An easy, soothing way to relieve itching is an oatmeal bath. Pour three cups of rolled oats or two cups of dried *Avena sativa* in a nylon stocking or a piece of cheesecloth and tie securely. If you have ground ginger, dried lavender, or slippery elm, add one-half cup to the oat sachet. These herbs soothe the nervous system and help prevent itching. Drop the sachet into the bathtub while you draw a hot bath. Wait twenty minutes, or until the water is the appropriate temperature, before letting your child soak in the tub. Or, use one to three drops of the essential oil of lavender or tea tree in the bath instead of oats or herbs.

Some other herbal remedies for chicken pox include burdock, red clover, and valerian, taken in tea or tincture form. Burdock and red clover soothe and cleanse the skin; valerian relaxes the nervous system and lessens the need to scratch. One or two cups of tea a day made with any of these herbs is an appropriate dose for kids younger than six years of age. Older kids may drink two or three cups per day. If you're using the tincture form of the herbs, follow the dosage on the bottle or Clark's rule (page 64).

COLD CARE

Colds are tricky little viruses that thrive on cold weather and dry air. Although not a serious illness, a cold can develop into a secondary infection of the lungs or sinuses if your child can't rest or if his immune system is depressed in some way. Although there is no cure for the common cold, there are natural ways to make your child more comfortable, ease his sore throat, quell his cough, and help him rest.

Offering liquids is important because a child with a cold can easily become dehydrated. Have him drink as much clear broth, juice, tea, and water as he can. Most kids love warm, homemade lemonade, which contains vitamin C and is easy to make. Squeeze the juice from half a lemon into a glass of room-temperature water and add one teaspoon honey (if the child is age two or older). You can also add a small piece of fresh garlic or a sprig of mint.

Diet also is important. Good foods to fight colds include blueberries, carob, carrots, and raspberries. These foods contain complex sugars called oligosaccharides that help prevent harmful bacteria from settling in the intestinal lining and may help prevent diarrhea that sometimes comes with a cold.

Garlic is the great herbal antibiotic, so increase your family's garlic intake throughout the cold season and especially during a family cold outbreak. If what you're cooking for dinner calls for garlic, increase the amount. Add garlic to clear broths, dice raw garlic for salad dressing, and roast garlic to smear on bread or add to pasta or mashed potatoes.

Oregano, long overlooked for its medicinal properties, contains more than thirty biologically active components, including antiviral properties. Use fresh or dried oregano on pastas, salads, and vegetables, and even in teas and baths.

For children who have a cold, an herbal bath can be soothing and therapeutic. To one or two quarts of boiling water, add one cup of a mixture of the following herbs: calendula, chamomile, lavender, and rosemary. Steep the mixture until it has cooled completely, strain the mixture and discard the herbs, and add the liquid to the bath water.

For vaporization, add a few drops of the eucalyptus, lavender, rosemary, or tea tree essential oil to a pot of boiling water. The steam will release the essential oil into the room.

Throughout cold season, practice good hygiene around the home. Clean doorknobs, faucets, toilet handles, toilet seats, and other frequently touched surfaces with essential oils of lavender, rosemary, peppermint, or tea tree. Frequent hand washing is important; soap and water work fine. There's no need for hand sanitizers or the like unless you're on the go.

For a burst of vitamin C, give your child Rose Hips Tea (page 141) or Rose Hips Fruit Leather (page 140). For a daily nutrition boost, try Family Vitamin-and-Mineral Powder (page 138).

Coughs

Look for teas, children's cough syrups, and cough drops that contain any of the following herbs: coltsfolt, echinacea, elderberry, garlic, lemon, mullein, oregano, peppermint, red clover, rose hips, sage, stinging nettle, thyme, and wild cherry bark. Homemade remedies include Cough and Throat Drops (page 148), Lemon Cough Syrup (page 150), Elderberry Cough Syrup (page 149), Vermont Cough Syrup (page 151), and Wild Cherry Cough Syrup (page 152).

Fever

At the onset of a fever, give five drops of echinacea tincture in juice or water (or just squirt it into the mouth if the child doesn't mind the taste) every three to four hours. If there is no change in the fever after thirty minutes, give five more drops. Repeat after another thirty minutes. (See What Constitutes Fever? and fever remedies, page 87.)

For children older than two years of age, prepare a tea. To five cups of boiling water, add one teaspoon *each* of the following herbs: catnip, chamomile, elder, lemon balm, and peppermint. Steep the tea until it is lukewarm, strain the tea, and discard the herbs. Give the child one-half cup of the tea three or four times a day.

Headache

Headaches associated with colds can be caused by fever and congestion. Sometimes dehydration can cause a headache, and a glass of water or juice could remedy the ache. A compress is very comforting for a headache—especially one made with essential oil of eucalyptus, lavender, lemon, peppermint, or rosemary.

Teas made from catnip, passionflower, rosemary, skullcap, or valerian can ease a headache. These herbs have relaxing and antianxiety effects, and valerian also promotes sleep. Try Headache Tea (page 159) or Headache Tincture (page 159). Children younger than ten years of age should not be given passionflower remedies, however.

Sinus Congestion

Fill your bathroom with steam from a hot shower. Add a few drops of essential oil, such as eucalyptus, lavender, or tea tree, to the water and let your child breathe in the steam and vapor. Gently massage her face with a warm, damp washcloth. If this is too painful, just continue with the steam. Painful sinuses could mean an infection. Check with your doctor or health-care practitioner.

When buying prepared remedies for sinus congestion, look for products such as easy-breathe teas and herbal vapor rubs that are especially formulated for sinus congestion. These can contain eucalyptus, garlic, horseradish, mustard, or onions. If your child runs away at the mere suggestion of any of those ingredients, try Garlic Honey (page 169), Sinus Tea for Kiddos (page 170), Super Sinus-Clearing Tea (page 169), or Echinacea Sinus Tea (page 170). (Horseradish should not be given to children younger than age four. Children under the age of six years should not use this herb medicinally.)

For information about sinus infection remedies, see page 93. This section includes instructions on how to use a neti pot, which can be helpful in treating sinus congestion.

Sneezing

The nose works as an air purifier for the lungs, cleaning inhaled air of bacteria and particles. When viruses and bacteria multiply in your nose during a cold, when a cloud of dust blows in your face, or when you have an allergic reaction, the nerve endings in the nose become irritated. With a blast of air, the nose sweeps its passageways clean.

Sneezing is a way for the body to rid itself of germs and clear the nasal passages. It's a good thing, even though it can be annoying.

Sore Throat

Sometimes it's hard to tell if your child has a sore throat, particularly if he's very young, unless you can get a good look at the throat. Hoarseness of the voice or a husky cry might also indicate a sore throat.

When buying herbal remedies for infants, look for products that are made specifically for infant use and contain mullein, rose hips, sage, or thyme. For older children, use drops, soothing teas, syrups, and throat sprays. Try Slippery Elm Cough Drops (page 176).

Inhalation Therapy

Steam inhalation using essential oils can be an effective way to clear a stuffy nose and head or ease a headache or allergies. Depending on the essential oils you use, steam inhalation can also calm the mind, nervous system, and spirit of older kids. However, because steam can burn and is potentially dangerous to children, steam inhalation therapy should be done only with adult supervision.

One simple technique is to put a few drops of essential oil on a washcloth and place it on the floor of the shower. The vapors will rise with the steam as the child showers. Alternatively, pour boiling water into a large bowl and add a few drops of essential oil. Drape a towel over your child's head, forming a tent over the steaming bowl, and have the child inhale the vapors through the nose a few times.

Older kids who tend to get sore throats or tonsillitis often benefit from gargling two or three times a day with warm water mixed with goldenseal tincture. To determine the dosage of tincture, follow Clark's rule (see page 64). Older kids who have a sore throat or laryngitis can gargle with warm saltwater (made with sea salt) or infusion of usnea or goldenseal, or equal parts infusion of red sage and chamomile. They also may benefit from gargling with teas prepared with the following herbs: blackberry leaves, elder flowers, red raspberry leaves, sage, or yarrow. In addition, older children can chew a small piece of osha root, which contains compounds that promote immunity and break infection.

Another good throat soother is a mixture of equal amounts of honey and apple cider vinegar, stirred or shaken well. Give one tablespoon as often as necessary to cut mucus in the throat.

Stuffy Nose

You can remove mucus from a baby's or a toddler's nose with a bulb syringe. Use saline nose drops from the pharmacy, or make your own. With a dropper, place two or three drops into one nostril at a time, then suction out the mucus with a bulb syringe. This is most effective when done before feedings, at naptime, and at bedtime.

COLIC

For parents, colic can be one of the most trying childhood ailments because it makes a baby cry for hours, seemingly for no reason. All babies cry, but a baby with colic does not respond to gestures of comfort, even when she is fed, loved, and has a dry diaper. If your baby cries at the same time every day and nothing you do seems to comfort her, she may have colic.

Colic is defined as crying for more than three hours per day, for at least three days a week, for more than three weeks at a time, in a baby who is otherwise well nourished and healthy. This condition usually starts a few weeks after birth and improves by age three months. That means a lot of long, loud nights for parents.

The causes of colic are unknown. My generation of parents was taught that colic indicated digestive problems. Although painful gas might contribute to colic, there is little evidence to prove that colic is linked to the digestive tract. Lactose intolerance has also been identified as a possible contributing factor, but that evidence is limited as well. An infant's temperament may also be a factor. A baby may be highly sensitive to her environment, and she may react to normal stimulation or changes by crying. Exposure to cigarette smoke may be another factor. Of course, no one should smoke around an infant at any time.

A parent can do several simple things to avoid or alleviate colic, such as slowing down feedings. If you are nursing, make sure the baby is properly latched onto the breast and isn't swallowing air unnecessarily. Give your baby homeopathic colic liquids or tablets, which are soft and dissolve in the baby's mouth. Sit your baby on your lap and gently and rhythmically pat her bottom or back. The rhythm and release of gas often help to soothe colic. Walking and gently bouncing the baby can also help, as can rocking or car rides. Some babies are comforted by music, singing, and chanting or white noise or wave machines.

Several teas for colicky babies are available in natural-food stores. They are made with tummy-soothing herbs, such as dill, fennel, ginger, and peppermint. Give no more than six tablespoons per day, one to two tablespoons at a time. Homemade fennel seed tea usually relieves a baby's gassy tummy. To make the tea, pour one cup of boiling water over one or two teaspoons of slightly crushed fennel seeds.

Detox for Children?

I'm often asked what I recommend as a good cleansing herb for children. My answer is an emphatic *nothing.* I don't believe in cleansing children's systems.

Cleansing generally means to flush or clear toxins from the body. This process often involves laxative herbs that are too harsh for children. Cleansing is uncomfortable for the child (and the parent), and it can lead to dehydration, which can result in fever and illness.

Children's health problems are generally related to environment and diet, so when parents ask about cleansing, I recommend that they take a look at what the child is eating. Children should be nourished rather than cleansed. To nourish them, we must add more high-quality foods and nutrients to our children's diets. In addition to a diet full of wholesome fruits, vegetables, and seeds, some herbal infusions can be particularly nourishing. These include alfalfa, dandelion leaf, oats, and stinging nettle taken two or three times a day. If the child is constipated, eating fresh fruit or pumpkin seeds and drinking more water can help.

Steep the tea for ten to fifteen minutes. Infants can be given one to three teaspoons of the tea for gas and colic. Usually one dose before bedtime is enough, but you can give it two to three times a day if necessary. Also, see recipes for Gripe Water Teas (pages 142–144), Catnip Tea (page 142), and Basil Tea (page 142).

Another way to comfort a colicky baby is to swaddle her in a blanket. Infants love this. It reminds them of the security of the womb and helps to keep them from being disturbed by their natural startle reflex. To wrap your infant, lay a blanket on a flat surface and fold down the top right corner about six inches. Place the baby on the blanket on her back with her head on the fold. Pull the corner near your baby's left hand across her body and tuck the edge under her right arm and her back. Bring the bottom corner up under the baby's chin, then bring the remaining corner over the baby's right arm and tuck the edge under her back on her left side. If your baby prefers to have her arms free, swaddle the baby under her arms. The football hold may also be comforting—position the baby on her tummy along the underside of your forearm with her head in the crook of your arm and her feet over your hands.

CONJUNCTIVITIS

lso known as pink eye, conjunctivitis is an inflammation of the conjunctiva, the lining that covers the back of the eyelid and part of the white of the eye. Bacteria, a virus, an allergy, or an adverse reaction can cause the inflammation. Eyes appear swollen and red, and they feel itchy and irritated. There may be a sticky discharge, and the child may not be able to open the affected eye in the morning when he wakes up. If pain, swollen lymph glands, or blurred vision are present, seek help from your doctor or health-care practitioner immediately.

Conjunctivitis is short-lived and easy to treat. Unfortunately, it is highly contagious and can whip through a family, classroom, or day-care center like the wind. During an outbreak, wash laundry in hot water and encourage frequent hand washing for the whole family.

Popular homeopathic eye drops are readily available in drug-stores, natural-food stores, and some supermarkets. These usually work well; however, if the eye hasn't healed in four days, contact your doctor or health-care practitioner.

Teas made from calendula, eyebright, goldenseal, lady's mantle, meadowsweet, and red raspberry leaf are effective eyewashes for kids with conjunctivitis. In one cup of warm water, make a weak tea using a teabag containing one of these herbs and reserve the soaked teabag. Use cotton balls dipped in the tea to wash the child's eye. Older children can lie down for a while or go to bed with the reserved teabag (it should be soaked but not dripping) on the affected eye.

You can also make an eyewash or eye compress with a strong tea or infusion. Use an eyecup or pour the cooled infusion over the affected eye. If using a compress, soak a clean cloth in the cooled infusion and apply it to the eye for ten minutes (or however long the child will sit still). Do not reuse the cloth. Use the eyewash or compress five or six times a day. Also, try any of the following eye-washes: Eyebright, Goldenseal, Purple Loosestrife, or Three-Flower (pages 145–147).

Other simple remedies for conjunctivitis include applying a fresh, cooling slice of cucumber to your child's eye or using a potato to make a compress. Potatoes contain anti-inflammatory properties that soothe the fragile skin around the eye. If the eyelids are swollen, make a compress of peeled, grated potato wrapped in clean cotton gauze. Apply the compress to the eye two or three times a day for ten minutes at a time. Also, if you happen to be breast-feeding, try squirting a little breast milk in the affected eye. Breast milk has antibiotic properties.

CONSTIPATION

Breast-fed infants rarely suffer from constipation. If you're dealing with constipation in a formula-fed baby, talk with your doctor to evaluate the situation and perhaps switch formulas. Constipation in children is usually a dietary issue, so I don't offer herbal remedies for it.

Simple diet modifications are usually all that's needed to fix constipation in children. Make sure your child is eating whole foods instead of processed ones: whole-grain bread instead of white bread, oatmeal from rolled oats instead of instant cereal, brown rice instead of white, and so on. In addition, offer lots of vegetables and fruits, especially apricots, peaches, pears, and prunes.

Psyllium seeds expand in water so they soften the stool and cleanse the intestines. The seeds are available at natural-food stores and can be mixed into smoothies, or sprinkled on cereal or a bowl of fruit and yogurt. For toddlers and children, begin with one teaspoon of psyllium per day. Increase to two teaspoons per day if necessary. Be sure, however, that your child drinks lots of water when taking psyllium; without the water, psyllium can actually make constipation worse.

In addition, exercise is important to keep bowels moving. Massage can also help: using almond or apricot kernel oil, gently rub your child's tummy in a clockwise direction.

Constipation Consternation

When your older child is constipated, consult a doctor if

- your child is experiencing pain, his stomach is distended, and he has no appetite; this could be a sign of a blockage or other intestinal problems;
- he has accidental bowel movements while not on the toilet;
- his bowel movements show signs of blood, either black or red; or
- withholding the bowel movement seems to be linked to emotional issues.

CRADLE CAP

Cradle cap will bother you more than it will bother your little one. Cradle cap is a condition in which the skin on the scalp (and sometimes beneath the eyebrows and behind the ears) produces excessive amounts of oil. The skin becomes bumpy, crusty, and scaly. Cradle cap is common in very young babies and eventually disappears on its own. But if you can't wait for that, there are several herbal remedies you can try.

With a cotton ball, apply olive oil or Cradle Cap Blend (page 153) to the scalp. (Do not use mineral oil or baby oil, which are both petroleum-based.) After an hour or so (or overnight), gently comb the baby's scalp to loosen the scales, or gently brush off the scales with a very soft toothbrush; then wash the head gently with a soft washcloth. You can also look for over-the-counter products that contain calendula, chamomile, or lavender. If cradle cap extends into the eye area or seems to be causing discomfort, consult your doctor or health-care practitioner.

CROUP

Croup is a viral infection that causes the lining of the airways, particularly the area just below the larynx, or voice box, to swell. Croup generally starts with cold symptoms and has a distinctive, seal-like barking cough that is usually worse at night.

For mild cases, keep a humidifier running. Alternatively, add ten drops of eucalyptus or peppermint essential oil to a vaporizer, or twenty drops to boiling water to make a vapor that is both relaxing and antibiotic. If your child has a serious case of croup and feels really miserable, take her into a hot, steamy bathroom; steam helps to loosen congestion.

If your child also has a fever, give echinacea tincture. For children ages two to four, give five drops of tincture in juice or warm water every three to four hours. For children ages five to ten, give fifteen drops in juice or warm water every three to four hours.

Chamomile relaxes the nervous system and helps relieve the aching chest caused by the coughing. Chamomile tea can be administered in small sips or by dropper two to three times a day. (The tea may be cooled to room temperature.) For a baby younger than one year, give one teaspoon or one dropper of tea two to three times a day. For toddlers ages one to two, give two teaspoons or two droppers of tea. For children ages three and older, give a half cup tea.

Call your doctor or health-care practitioner if your child exhibits any of the following symptoms in addition to the cold symptoms and barking cough:

- a belly that sinks in with breathing
- bluish or pale color around the mouth
- difficulty breathing or rapid breathing
- drooling or difficulty swallowing
- high fever (see What Constitutes Fever? page 87)
- inactivity
- skin between the ribs that pulls in with each breath
- stridor, a high-pitched, squeaky noise when the child exhales

CUTS AND SCRAPES

Cuts and scrapes are an everyday occurrence with kids, so it's a good idea to keep around some sort of herbal "heal-all" salve. Look for prepared salves or first-aid remedies that contain one or more of the following herbs: calendula, chickweed, comfrey, lavender, plantain, and St. John's wort. As an alternative, use any of these herbs singly or combine them to make infusions that can be used in compresses. Also, see Comfrey Compress (page 176), Garlic Honey (page 169), Soothing Salve (page 175), Plantain Salve (page 174), and First-Aid Remedy (page 161).

DIAPER RASH

One of new parents' most common worries is diaper rash. This red irritation is most usually caused by prolonged skin contact with a wet or soiled diaper. Other types of diaper rash, however, are caused by candida or bacteria. Breast-fed babies tend to have fewer diaper rashes because their urine and stool do not contain the substances in formula that cause rash.

The main treatment for diaper rash is to change diapers frequently. In addition, during every change, wash baby's diaper area with mild soap and water. Use a soft cloth—not chemical-laced baby wipes. I see much less diaper rash in babies who wear cloth diapers than in those who wear disposables. It's easy to tell when cloth diapers are wet, and parents change them quickly. In contrast, disposables contain layers of a gel that absorbs wetness, making it harder for parents to tell if the diaper is wet. This gel has been known to irritate the skin and even cause illness.

One of the best ways to prevent diaper rash is to not diaper at all. Some parents practice "elimination communication," in which they use signals and timing (and even intuition) to teach a baby to control urination and bowel movements. You can also simply let your baby "air out" frequently. (Babies love this, but make sure the room is warm with no drafts.)

Before you put on a clean diaper, you can smear on organic soybean (vegetable) shortening as a great barrier of protection or sprinkle on a plant-based baby powder, such as cornstarch. (Avoid talcum powders; talc has been linked to several cancers.) Also, try Bum-Bum Powder (page 153).

There are plenty of herb-based creams and salves on the market that work well for diaper rash. Look for products that contain calendula, plantain, or St. John's wort, all known for their skin-healing and rash-preventing properties. Or, try Taro's Bummi Cream (page 155), Jacob's Salve (page 154), Goldenseal Salve (page 154), or Plantain Salve (page 174) as both preventatives and curatives.

Candida or yeast infections look like diaper rashes gone terribly wrong. The classic signs of a candida diaper rash are little white bumps that "grow" on bright red skin. A good topical treatment for a candida rash is plain, organic yogurt without additives, fruit, or sugar. The live active cultures in the yogurt help reduce and kill the yeast. Once or twice a day, gently wash the diaper area with plain water and let the baby air-dry. Spread a small dollop of yogurt on the rash before putting on a clean, dry diaper (preferably cloth). You can also open an acidophilus capsule once or twice a day and sprinkle its contents over the baby's bum for the same effect.

DIARRHEA

The causes of diarrhea are many and varied, so much so that it can be difficult at times to determine what is actually causing a child's frequent, watery bowel movements. Another confounding factor, especially in breast-fed infants, is that their normal bowel movements are very soft. Sometimes it is simply difficult to tell if your baby has diarrhea. To be able to determine if you child has diarrhea, you must know what your child's healthy stool looks and smells like.

Babies can have up to ten bowel movements a day. However, it's not just the frequency of bowel movements but also the consistency (or water content) that defines diarrhea. Some things that can cause diarrhea in children are:

- a new food or brand of formula
- food allergies
- food poisoning
- infection by bacteria, cold viruses, or parasites
- medications, such as antibiotics
- switching from breast milk to formula and back again
- teething

Although many doctors say teething and diarrhea are unrelated, most parents would disagree. I think teething causes excess saliva to be produced and swallowed, adding liquid to the bowels.

Diarrhea can lead to dehydration. To avoid dehydration, make sure your child is drinking plenty of water, juice, and other liquids. Some signs of dehydration in children are:

- dry, cool, blotchy skin
- dry mouth and tongue
- fast and weak pulse
- fever
- few or no tears
- irritability
- muscle cramps
- rapid breathing
- sleepiness
- sunken eyes, cheeks, or fontanel

Nursing mothers can take infants to the breast more often to avoid dehydration. Studies have found that breast-feeding lowers the frequency and duration of diarrhea in infants younger than six months, and that breast milk protects against at least two types of bacterial diarrhea.

My favorite remedy for treating diarrhea in children is blackberry leaf tea, which is strong and highly astringent. I recommend it only for children two years of age and older. To make the tea, add two teaspoons of dried blackberry leaf tea to one cup of boiling water. Let the tea steep until cool. Give one-fourth to one-half cup to a toddler, three times per day. Older children may drink two to three cups of tea per day. Use blackberry leaf tea for only one or two days, and seek medical treatment if there's no change in that time.

Rice cooking water is another simple remedy for diarrhea. It is nourishing, contains soluble fiber, and is a great source of vitamin B. Make rice with extra water, and drain off and cool the water. Let your child drink as much as he wants.

Ginger tea is used in the developing world as a treatment for diarrhea produced by bacteria. There are many prepared ginger teas on the market. Or, try Homemade Ginger Tea (page 156). Give one to two teaspoons of cooled ginger tea to an infant two or three times a day; give a toddler two to four tablespoons two to three times a day; and give older kids one to three cups a day.

Candied or crystallized ginger can help tummy and intestinal problems. Let your child have two or three candies once or twice a day. Slippery Elm Gruel (page 156) is also beneficial because it soothes and nourishes the intestinal tract.

Important: If you think your child's diarrhea may be from food poisoning or if your child is severely dehydrated, consult your doctor or health-care practitioner immediately.

EAR INFECTIONS

By the age of six, almost 95 percent of all children will have had otitis media, or a middle ear infection. Ear infections are more common in children than in adults because children's eustachian tubes are smaller and more horizontal, which hampers drainage. Middle ear infections occur because of an infection by a bacteria or a virus, usually as a result of a cold. Inflammation causes pus, which presses on the eardrum, causing great pain. Chronic infections may occur when the eustachian tube becomes persistently blocked due to repeated ear infections, allergies, adenoid problems, or some sort of trauma to the ear.

Persistent ear infections may lead to a ruptured eardrum and eventual hearing loss. Doctors prescribe antibiotics for ear infections because they kill the bacteria and can prevent the infection from spreading to the brain or the bone around the ears. Kids generally will feel better faster when they are given antibiotics. However, research indicates that most simple ear infections can clear up on their own within four to seven days, although the child will be feverish and in pain during that time.

How can you tell if your child has a middle ear infection? Ear infections are almost always preceded by a cold with a runny nose. Older children, of course, can tell you their ears hurt. Little ones, though, will suddenly become very fussy, day or night, and wake up more often at night. They also will have a low-grade fever, not much appetite, and may or may not tug at their ears. It may be uncomfortable for them to lie flat. Blood or pus may drain from their ears if their eardrums have ruptured. (Ruptured eardrums almost always heal just fine. In fact, a child will feel some relief after the eardrums have ruptured and the pressure is released.)

Important: Do not administer remedies if you suspect your child's eardrum has perforated. Contact your doctor or health-care practitioner.

Several brands of drops specifically for ear pain are available in natural-food stores. Look for herbal products that contain garlic, mullein, and St. John's wort. Garlic and mullein oils have antibiotic properties that fight ear infection. Studies have shown that drops containing St. John's wort are more effective in stopping ear pain than standard painkilling ear drops.

You can make your own ear drop oil blend of garlic, mullein, and St. John's wort (see Achy Ear Oil, page 157). Or, add two drops of tea tree essential oil to one tablespoon of olive oil and mix well. Use one or two drops in the affected ear two to three times a day.

In addition to the eardrops, give your child echinacea tincture to boost her immune system. If there is no children's dosage on the package, give half the adult dose to children ages six to thirteen years, and one-quarter the adult dose to children age six years and under. For an infant younger than two years, use one to two drops. Give the echinacea in water or juice, or straight if your child will take it that way.

In addition, the following can help when your child has an ear infection: Give your child hot, fresh lemonade or ginger tea, which are warming and soothing. Run the humidifier at night to moisten and soothe membranes. And, if you happen to be breast-feeding, try squirting a little breast milk, which has antibiotic properties, in each ear.

ECZEMA

E czema is a generic term for acute or chronic inflammation of the skin. It can look as benign as a pinkish-red rash, or it can be crusty, itchy, oozing, painful, and scaly—or a combination of these. Difficult cases can cause scarring or darkening of the skin. Eczema can plague children, and their parents, for months or years.

The cause of eczema can be a mystery. It can stem from allergic reactions to animal dander, foods, laundry detergent, lotions, soaps, synthetic fabrics—the list seems endless. One mom I know finally narrowed the cause of her son's severe eczema to the carpet fiber in their new house.

Eczema that appears under the arms, on the undersides of the wrists, in the crooks of the arms, and on the backs of the knees is a classic sign of food allergy. (Breast-fed babies can have allergic reactions to foods consumed by their mothers.) If your child has eczema in these areas, particularly within one or two hours after eating, consult your doctor or health-care practitioner about possible food allergies. You may want to ask your doctor or an allergist about an elimination diet, which removes highly allergenic foods from the diet for a couple of weeks and reintroduces them one at a time over a week or two. If your child has an eczema flare-up an hour or two after eating the reintroduced food, he may be allergic to it. Foods that are considered highly allergenic include dairy products, eggs, fish, nuts (especially peanuts), shellfish, soy, strawberries, and wheat.

I have worked with children whose eczema covered 70 percent of the body. Almost miraculous healing resulted when they drank red clover tea and bathed daily in water mixed with a gallon of red clover tea. To make red clover tea, add one teaspoon of dried red clover to one cup of boiling water. Let the tea steep ten or fifteen minutes, until cooled. Give your child the tea two to three times a day. An infant may be given two tablespoons; a toddler, four to five tablespoons; a child, one-half to one cup; and a teen, up to three cups. For spot breakouts, apply a soaked tea bag.

You can also give red clover tincture two to three times a day. An infant may be given two to three drops; a toddler, five to ten drops; a child, ten to fifteen drops; and a teen, twenty to thirty drops. Another option is to give your child tinctures of burdock, chickweed, cleavers, or echinacea internally two to three times a day. An infant may be given two drops; a toddler, five to ten drops; older children, ten to twelve drops; and teens, fifteen to twenty drops.

Some helpful herbs that can be taken as teas or infusions include burdock, lavender, lemon balm, milky oats, plantain, red clover, and stinging nettle. Or, try Eczema Tea (page 158). Infants may be given two to three tablespoons per day; toddlers, up to one cup; older children, two cups; and teenagers, two to three cups.

Another eczema remedy is to apply flaxseed oil to the rash. (If you can't find flaxseed oil in a bottle, make a hole in a flaxseed oil capsule and squeeze the oil onto the skin.) In addition, give your child flaxseeds or flaxseed oil each day to help balance his fatty acid intake, which has been shown to improve eczema. Older children can take up to one or two flaxseed capsules or up to two tablespoons of flaxseed oil per day. Children ages two to twelve can have up to one teaspoon of ground flaxseeds or one teaspoon of fresh flaxseed oil daily. For their infants' benefit, breast-feeding mothers can take one or two flaxseed capsules or one or two tablespoons of flaxseed oil per day.

Most traditional treatments for eczema focus on alleviating the symptoms. I usually suggest topical applications for eczema. If you are buying a prepared herbal salve, look for one that uses one of the following oils as its base: avocado, borage seed, evening primrose, jojoba, rose hip seed, sesame, sweet almond, or wheat germ. The salve can contain helpful herbs, such as calendula, comfrey, evening primrose, marshmallow, plantain, red clover, rose, rosemary, and sandalwood. Apply the salve freely to relieve itching and heal the skin.

Homemade eczema remedies, such as salves, can include oil infused with any of the following herbs: calendula, comfrey, plaintain, rose hips, and St. John's wort. A simple remedy is to add a pinch of dried goldenseal to a tablespoon of cream, and rub it on the rash. Or, try Goldenseal Salve (page 154), Plantain Salve (page 174), or Soothing Salve (page 175). You can also mix together equal parts of dried burdock root, marshmallow, yarrow, and yellow dock. In a small pot, add one heaping tablespoon of the herbs to one cup of boiling water. Let the tea simmer for twenty minutes, remove it from the heat, and let it cool. Use the tea as a compress or add it to a bath.

Parents should make sure children with eczema eat a wholesome diet and get sunshine and fresh air every day. They also can help by taking some household precautions. For your child's laundry, use a gentle, fragrance-free detergent or soap. Or try a natural product called "soap nuts," which are dried nuts (similar to lychee nuts) from the chinese soapberry tree (*Sapindus mukorrosi*) that have been used as laundry detergent in some Asian countries for centuries. Soap nuts actually are soapy due to their high saponin content. Do not use fabric softeners of any type. They leave a residue that may irritate a child's skin. Do not use soap for cleansing the skin. Instead, use a weak boric acid solution or a solution of one teaspoon of salt to one quart of water.

FEVER

Most fevers—those between 100 and 104 degrees Fahrenheit— are generally not that harmful. The majority are caused by viruses and may last three to five days.

Just because your child has a high fever does not mean he has a serious illness. How your child feels and acts should determine whether he needs medical attention. Ask your doctor for guidelines. In general, get medical attention if your child has a low-grade fever for a few hours or a fever over 102.5 degrees Fahrenheit.

What Constitutes Fever?

Fever has conventionally been defined as a rectal temperature over 100.4 degrees Fahrenheit or 38 degrees Celsius. Temperatures measured orally and auxiliary (in the armpit) are usually lower.

Fever itself generally is not life threatening unless it is extremely and persistently high, such as 107 degrees Fahrenheit (41.6 degrees Celsius) and higher when measured rectally. Seek immediate treatment when fever reaches 102 degrees Fahrenheit.

Give a tincture of any of the following herbs in juice or water every three to four hours: burdock, dandelion, echinacea, goldenseal, or yarrow. For infants age one year and younger, give one to two drops; for ages one to two years, two to four drops; for ages three to four years, four to six drops; and for ages eight to twelve years, ten to fifteen drops.

Make a tea by adding one teaspoon of dried parsley or red raspberry leaf to one cup of boiling water. Let the tea steep twenty minutes. Give it to your child three times a day. Infants may have three tablespoons; toddlers may have one-half cup; older children may have one cup; and teens, one to two cups.

For a healing bath, add four tablespoons of grated fresh ginger to warm bath water. The bath will open pores, promote perspiration, and flush out toxins.

HEAD LICE

Head lice are insect parasites that are found on the scalp. Infection with head lice is called pediculosis. It is no longer unusual for children to bring home head lice. If your child contracts lice, it does not mean that your family is unclean. Lice infestations sweep through schools and day-care centers like wildfire these days, and it can be a trial to get rid of them.

Suspect lice if your child is scratching her head madly and has red rashes on her scalp and the back of her neck. Look closely and you may see nits, tiny tear-drop-shape lice eggs, attached to individual hairs. The color of these nits may range from translucent (freshly laid) to brown (older and perhaps no longer viable).

Many natural-food stores sell natural products to combat head lice. Homemade herbal remedies for head lice are easy to make and simple to use. Try Mild Head Lice Oil (page 160) or Lice Leavers Oil (page 160).

After your child has been treated, reduce the chance of reinfestation by cleaning the house thoroughly. Vacuum furniture and rugs—everything. Wash the bedding and clothing in hot water and dry them on the hottest setting. Place the child's stuffed animals and pillows in the clothes dryer on the highest temperature setting for two hours. If any of these items can't go in the dryer, put them in sealed garbage bags and store them in the garage for three weeks. Finally, discard hair combs and brushes, and replace them with new ones.

INFLUENZA

Flu is essentially a severe cold with fever and body aches, and sometimes nausea and vomiting. Flu epidemics hit in late fall and early winter. Every year, the new flu strain is a little bit different from the previous year's version because it is caused by viruses that readily mutate or change. But generally, flu is an infection of the lungs and airways that starts with chills and fever and progresses to include runny nose, sore throat, cough, headache, muscle aches, weakness, and fatigue. Flu can be particularly hard on little children. Complications can include either viral or bacterial pneumonia.

Flu lasts two or three days, but it might take five days for the fever to normalize. The cough, however, can last ten days or more, and the chest irritation, fatigue, and weakness can go on for weeks. Your child can safely resume his normal activities twenty-four hours after his temperature goes down to normal.

Flu is mainly treated with lots of rest and fluids. Start pushing these as soon as symptoms begin. In addition, start herbal remedies that boost immunity right away. Give one-half teaspoon of an extract blend of equal parts of goldenseal and echinacea in juice or water every two hours to children older than six years of age. (Consult an herbalist for flu remedies for children younger than six years of age and infants.)

Herb teas that are helpful in treating flu include astragalus, boneset, echinacea, elderberry, ginger, and rose hips. Elderberry extract has been shown to relieve flu, cold, and sinus symptoms four days earlier than other medications. Look for herbal flu products for children that contain these herbs. Or, try Immunity Tonic Tea (page 139) or Immunity Tonic Tincture (page 140).

Support formulas, called tonics, that contain astragalus, dandelion, goldenseal, and licorice can be especially helpful during flu season because they provide nourishment, eliminate toxins, and destroy bacteria. Astragalus is available in chips that can be added to soups and broths, and the dried herb can be brewed as a tea that your child can drink once or twice a day. Dandelion provides potassium, stimulates kidney function, and acts as a diuretic. Goldenseal is known to help eliminate toxins and destroy bacteria.

Children who have the flu benefit from drinking hot liquids and eating nourishing, warm foods. Make hot soup and pots of hot tea for your child. Miso soup is healing and highly nutritious. Look for herbal and nutritional products for children that contain beta-carotene, vitamins A and C, and zinc. And serve foods such as broccoli, cantaloupe, carrots, oranges, pecans, pine nuts, strawberries, sweet potatoes, and wheat germ and bran.

It's important for children who have the flu to dress warmly and avoid drafts. Warm baths can also be comforting. Add one or two drops of essential oils of lavender or eucalyptus to bath water. Body massages can be relaxing for kids with flu. Try Cold and Flu Body Rub (page 138).

Change bed linens often to lessen the chance of spreading infection. Spritz bed sheets with lavender or rosemary spray for added disinfection. These herbs also help relax the child and keep nasal passages clear. Try Flu Preventer Children's Toy Cleaner (page 139) to help kill germs. It's also a good disinfectant for doorknobs, laundry areas, toilets, and other places that harbor flu germs.

HAND, FOOT, AND MOUTH DISEASE

Hand, foot, and mouth disease is a relatively common infection caused by a coxsackievirus. The first signs of infection are a sore throat and fever. Then sores appear in the mouth, and a rash develops on the palms of the hands, soles of the feet, and other places on the body (usually the trunk). Conventional medicine can suppress symptoms but can't cure the condition.

This disease is highly communicable, transmitted by touch, mucus, and coughing. Make sure your child washes his hands frequently and uses a clean tissue with each blow. Hands should be washed after contacting mucus, saliva, or any other bodily fluids.

Avoid giving your child highly acidic foods and drinks, such as citrus fruits, because the acid will sting and aggravate the mouth sores. Saltwater rinses can soothe the mouth sores and sore throat. Use one-half teaspoon of sea salt in one glass of hot water. Let the saltwater sit until it cools to room temperature and is completely dissolved.

Another great remedy for mouth sores is a rinse with calendula tea, or twenty drops of calendula tincture in one-half cup of water. Myrrh, sage, and yarrow tinctures will also work since these herbs are astringents that aid the healing process. Any of these herbs can be used to make cooled tea to be used as a gargle. In addition, chamomile, lavender, or lemon balm teas can be used for their soothing effects.

For the rash, try the same baths that are recommended for chicken pox (page 70). You can also use olive oil or infused herbal oils with calendula, lavender, St. John's wort, or plantain. Or, try the antibiotic-type gel, Anti-Gel (page 158).

MUSCLE ACHES AND PAINS

K ids can have sore muscles, too. They play hard. Older kids may be in sports programs that require them to use muscles they might not have been using lately. Like adults, they need something to ease the aches.

Look for products that contain herbs such as arnica, meadow-sweet, oats, skullcap, and St. John's wort. These can be found in teas, tinctures, and topical treatments. Also, keep Muscle-Easing Liniment (page 168) on hand.

WHOOPING COUGH (PERTUSSIS)

W hooping cough is a highly contagious infection of the respiratory system caused by a strain of bacteria called *Bordetella pertussis*. Most children are immunized against the disease at an early age; however, some children are beginning to contract whooping cough ten years or so after their vaccinations. The U.S. Centers for Disease Control report that the disease is on the rise, particularly in children between the ages of ten and nineteen.

Whooping cough begins as an innocuous cold, with sneezing, runny nose, and a general malaise that can last up to two weeks. But then the coughing starts. The child will have fits of coughing with a distinctive inhalation that makes a high-pitched "whooping" sound (thus the name). Infected children cough up volumes of thick mucus and may cough so hard they vomit. Infants may choke, stop breathing, and turn blue. Coughing comes in spasms, with one quickly following another. The disease and coughing fits subside in about six weeks; however, the cough may linger for weeks or even months.

Older kids are generally treated at home. Whooping cough can be more severe in infants, however, and they usually must be hospitalized and given mechanical breathing assistance, oxygen, and IV fluids. Brain damage and retardation due to bleeding and swelling of the brain are rare. About two percent of children die from the disease; most of them are one year of age or younger.

Cough medicines are not generally effective for whooping cough, so they're usually not recommended. It is also unclear whether antibiotics do much. They may shorten the infectious period if started in time, but they probably do little to affect the outcome of the disease.

Look for herbal remedies that include licorice root, sundew, or thyme. Sundew is a well-known herbal remedy for whooping cough because it's a powerful bronchial antispasmodic and antitussive. Licorice root is a demulcent and expectorant that helps move phlegm; it also is an anti-inflammatory. Thyme, another traditional whooping cough treatment, has antibacterial, expectorant, and antispasmodic properties. Teas made with these herbs can help. However, because children who have whooping cough have a strong cough reflex and tend to vomit, teas might not stay down long enough to take effect.

There are a couple of over-the-counter "herbal tussin" products on the market you can try for the coughing. Or, try Super-Cough Tea (page 180) and Cough-Stop Tea (page 179).

ROSEOLA

Roseola is a viral infection that usually affects little ones between the ages of six months and two years. It begins with a respiratory infection, lack of appetite, and a high fever. A fine, red rash will appear on the neck, face, arms, and legs. The rash's spots will blanch when you touch them, and some individual spots may have a lighter "halo" around them.

Call your doctor if your child is lethargic or not drinking liquids, and if you can't get the fever to stay down. (See What Constitutes Fever? and fever remedies, page 88.). In about 10 to 15 percent of children with roseola, a very high fever will cause febrile seizures. A baby may become unconscious, jerk or twitch for two to three minutes, and lose bladder or bowel control. If this happens, seek emergency care immediately.

Oatmeal baths can soothe the rash (see page 70). You can also add one or two drops of lavender essential oil to the bath to soothe any itching or soreness associated with the rash.

SINUS INFECTIONS

Sinus infections result in congestion and pounding headaches that can progress to coughing and fever. In some children, a sinus infection can lead to a systemic infection and dehydration if not treated. If your child's face on either side of the nose or above the nose is painful to the touch, she probably has a sinus infection. If she is too ill to engage in her normal activities and play, consult your doctor or health-care practitioner.

Look for herbal remedies that are specially formulated for sinus and allergy problems and herbal teas that contain elder flowers, hibiscus, rose hips, sage, or thyme. Or, try Sinus Extract Blend (page 171), Super Sinus-Clearing Tea (page 169), Echinacea Sinus Tea (page 170), or Sinus Mustard (page 173) to open sinus passages. To boost immunity and fight infection, use extracts of astragalus, echinacea, or goldenseal in water or juice two to three times a day.

Diet is important for a child who has a sinus infection: Make sure your child gets enough vitamins A and C and zinc. Omit dairy products and wheat to slow mucus production. And clear your child's system with drinks such as diluted fruit juices and hot lemonade.

Steam treatments can be beneficial. Turn on the shower, close the drain, and add a few drops of essential oil, such as eucalyptus, lavender, pine, or tea tree, to the water. Fill your bathroom with steam, and let your child breathe in the steam and vapor. Or, use lavender bath salts for a soothing bath. See Shower Soother (page 171) and Sinus Headache Bath Salts (page 172).

Gently massage your child's face with a warm, damp washcloth. You can also make a massage oil by combining one drop of lavender or eucalyptus essential oil and one tablespoon of olive oil or apricot kernel oil. If your child finds massage too painful, just continue with the steam treatments. For a soothing rest, try a Sinus Headache Pillow (page 172).

Using a Neti Pot

If your older child often has sinus congestion and sinus infections, consider teaching her how to use a neti pot for regular sinus irrigation and cleansing. A neti pot is a small, almost teapot-shape pot that is filled with lukewarm saltwater. Your child should put the pot's spout in one nostril and pour the water into the nostril, letting it drain through the sinuses and out the other nostril. You can buy neti pots in drugstores, health-food stores, and online.

Most neti pots come with instructions; use them as directed. The important thing to remember is to use saltwater. Using water out of the tap without added salt can cause painful stinging. The salt used in the neti pot should contain no chemicals or anticaking agents and should be free of iodine. Sea salt, kosher salt, or pharmaceutical-grade salt are all good choices.

Have your child use the neti pot once or twice a week to cut down on sinus congestion and infections. Neti pots are also useful for kids who have allergies or get a lot of colds.

SPRAINS

A sprain means a ligament has been stretched or torn. Many herbs can be beneficial in treating sprains when used topically as compresses, oils, and soaks. These include arnica, comfrey, ginger, oats, plantain, and St. John's wort. See Comfrey Compress (page 176). Salves and ointments can also offer relief. Look for products that contain arnica, chickweed, clove, comfrey, marjoram, plantain, and St. John's wort.

Internal remedies can be helpful in treating sprains. Look for products that contain chickweed, horsetail, oats, plantain, and stinging nettle.

TEETHING

A baby's first tooth usually appears before six months of age, although many babies get teeth much earlier. By age three, babies have a complete set of twenty teeth. From the time the first tooth emerges until the set is complete, parents can expect some fussy days. Your baby could be teething if she cries during nursing; is drooling, grumpy, and unsettled; and maybe even has a slight fever (below 100 degrees Fahrenheit). Check for red and tender gums.

Teething babies love to chew on just about anything and everything, including frozen cloth. Wet a clean terry cloth washcloth, wring it well, fold it, wrap it in a plastic sandwich bag, and freeze. You can also let your baby chew on a piece of cleaned licorice root. (Discard the root when it starts to fray.) Licorice will offer relief, and the root is firm enough to gnaw on.

Look for herbal teething oils at your market. I also highly recommend homeopathic teething tablets. They're soft, dissolve instantly, and are easy to use, so keep them on hand. For homemade remedies to soothe the gums, see Baby Gumming Rub (page 178), Slippery Elm Paste (page 179), and Peppermint Rub (page 178).

THRUSH

T hrush, or candidiasis, is a fungal infection of the mouth that is usually caused by *Candida albicans*. The infection forms patchy, white spots or a white film over the inside of the mouth. It usually coats the tongue, irritates the gums, and can be quite painful, particularly for babies as they nurse.

Candida normally lives harmlessly on the skin, in the mouth, in the intestinal tract, and in the vagina. It is usually kept in check by other bacteria and microorganisms in the body. However, several factors can cause an overgrowth, which leads to infection. These include antibiotic use; hot, humid weather; illness; immune system disorders; poor hygiene; and tight clothing.

In young children and babies, candida overgrowth can result in thrush and severe diaper rash (see page 80). An effective remedy for thrush is gentian violet, which can be purchased at a pharmacy. (You do not need a prescription for it; however, you may not find it on the shelves and may need to ask the pharmacist for it.) To use gentian violet, moisten a cotton swab with one drop and apply it inside the baby's mouth once a day for three or four days. A sweet side effect is your baby's cute, purple smile.

Another simple remedy for candida is plain, organic yogurt without additives, fruit, or sugar. Read the label to make sure the yogurt contains bifidobacterium or lactobacillus. These bacteria do not eradicate thrush. They do, however, help keep it within healthful levels. Swab your baby's mouth with yogurt twice a day or, for the same effect, sprinkle acidophilus powder on the affected area.

Make sure anything that comes into contact with the infection is sterilized or washed in hot water: bras, breast pads, breast pump parts, breast shields, diapers, pacifiers, teethers, toothbrushes, toys, and underwear. If you breast-feed, use the same remedies as your baby—treat your nipples with the gentian violet or plain yogurt.

WARTS

Common warts are, well, common in children. They are caused by several varieties of papillomavirus and generally don't itch or cause any pain unless they're in an uncomfortable or awkward location. Warts are highly contagious, so picking at them or even touching them can make them spread.

My youngest son went through a warty phase. He had two on his fingers that really bugged him. We rubbed the sap from the greater celandine plant on his warts twice a day, and they were gone within a week. (Just break the stem or remove the leaves, and the sap will ooze out. Merely rub the sap on the wart, which will stain yellow.) When the warts came back the following year, we repeated the treatment with the same results.

Common warts generally disappear on their own within a year. However, you can try some simple herbal remedies to speed up the process: Rub one drop of tea tree essential oil on the wart daily. Apply infusion of thuja, which can be made by combining one teaspoon dried thuja with one cup of boiling water. With a cotton ball, apply the cooled infusion to the wart three or four times a day. Or soak cotton gauze in castor oil. Apply the gauze each night before bed, and leave it on overnight. Continue until the wart has disappeared.

ESPECIALLY FOR TEENS

Teenagers have their own set of health concerns, including acne, oily and problem skin, and, for teen girls, menstrual problems.

Acne

Teens can be volatile in personality, and their skin problems can be volatile as well. Teens grow quickly and should lead active, healthy, and vital lives. Unfortunately, teens who have acne can be subject to social stigmas. One way parents can help is to nourish them with whole foods, vitamins, and a little herbal help when needed. Herbal remedies for acne are entirely preferable to the harsh chemicals, stinging astringents, and antibiotics that constitute traditional acne treatment.

Affecting 85 percent of all people some time during their teen years, acne is a disease of the hair follicle and sebaceous glands of the face, neck, chest, back, and upper arms. It is triggered by increased amounts of male hormones, called androgens, that surge in both boys and girls during puberty. Androgens cause an increased secretion of sebum and enlarged pores; bacteria cause the inflammations that lead to pimples.

One of the first favors you can do for a teen with acne is to make sure he's drinking lots of water and eating a diet high in fiber and loaded with fruits and vegetables (preferably raw), whole grains, bran, and other complex carbohydrates. (See Foods and Drinks for Good Skin, page 98.) Among other things, these foods help keep the digestive tract moving so the skin is not burdened by wastes it can't handle.

Some teens notice that certain foods aggravate their acne, while others don't notice any effects from food. (See Foods and Drinks to Avoid, page 98.) Studies have linked acne with dairy products and sugar. Some acne has been shown to develop because of an allergic reaction to dairy products. Encourage your teen to avoid dairy foods for a month and see if the acne improves, then gradually reintroduce dairy products to see if the condition worsens.

Proper skin care involves gentle yet effective cleansing. Drugstore shelves—and television commercials—are filled with harsh acne cleansers, soaps, treatments, and washes. These can be unnecessary. Often, all a teen needs is a rinse with plain water. If you and your teen think more is needed, look for herbal skin cleansers that are formulated specifically for acne. Many health-food stores sell excellent herbal skin-care cleansers, masks, moisturizers, scrubs, and toners. I suggest a mask or a scrub once a week. Try Muddy Mask (page 133), Easy-Does-It Scrub (page 131), and Goddess Face Scrub (page 132).

Skin lotions, toners, and washes are designed to cleanse the skin and shrink the pores. Buy toners that are based on lavender, lemon, rose, or witch hazel. Or, try some of the acne remedies in chapter 6.

After washing her face, your teen should gently pat her skin dry. Rubbing it roughly with a towel can be too harsh. If your teen uses toner, make sure she does not rub her face when applying it. Patting fresh lemon juice onto the skin twice a day can also be a good habit. Finally, be sure your teen shampoos her hair frequently.

When purchasing herbal remedies for acne, look for products that contain gentle essential oils, such as lavender and tea tree, and ingredients such as calendula, chamomile, chickweed, fennel, green tea, lemon,

Foods and Drinks for Good Skin

apricots

broccoli

carrots

celery

cucumber

fruit

garlic

green vegetables (including kale)

kelp

onions

peaches

seaweed

sprouts

squash

sweet potato

vegetable juice

watercress

whole grains

Foods and Drinks to Avoid

alcohol

caffeinated drinks

chocolate

citrus (except lemon juice)

dairy products

eggs

fried foods and other fatty foods

meat (including fish and poultry)

nut butters

processed or refined foods

sugar

wheat

plantain, rose petals, and witch hazel. Other acne-fighting herbs found in over-the-counter herbal preparations include bergamot, burdock, comfrey, cypress, geranium, helichrysum, jojoba, plantain, red clover, rosemary, and rosewood.

Menstrual Problems

Painful Periods

Pain during menstrual periods is of two types: primary dysmenorrhea and secondary dysmenorrhea. The first type is caused by prostaglandins, chemical compounds that, among other things, have hormonal effects that cause uterine cramping. Some cramping and symptoms such as backache, diarrhea, headache, and nausea are pretty normal and are to be expected during the first couple of days of a teen's menstrual cycle. However, if pain and other symptoms are so severe that they keep your daughter from her normal activities, consult your doctor or health-care practitioner. She could have secondary dysmenorrhea, which is pain caused by a physical problem, such as endometriosis, fibroids, hormonal imbalance, pelvic inflammatory disease, polyps, or other conditions.

Diet is key. To ease pain during her periods, your teen should eat a balanced diet with lots of fruits and vegetables, stay away from caffeine to reduce any jitters, and reduce her salt and sodium intake to help minimize bloating.

Girls who have crampy periods should begin a lifetime diet that includes a lot of calcium and calcium-rich foods. Calcium is necessary for muscle contraction; in supplements, it is often paired with magnesium, which is essential for muscle relaxation. Without adequate calcium, muscles cramp more easily, resulting in more painful menstrual cramps. The suggested calcium intake for teen girls is 800 milligrams per day, which can be attained through calcium supplements or calcium-rich foods, such as dark green, leafy vegetables; soy foods; and yogurt. Other good sources include almonds, almond butter, black-strap molasses, broccoli, collard and mustard greens, figs, fortified rice and soymilk, kale, seaweed, and tahini. It's especially important for a girl to eat these foods about a week and a half before her period is expected to begin.

Exercise and reducing stress have also been shown to reduce painful periods. Make sure your daughter stays active and finds time to decompress from the school and social demands that press on young girls.

Warm baths, warm sitz baths, and heating pads help keep the body warm, which also helps to ease the cramping. Pour one-half cup witch hazel or white oak bark tincture into the bath water to help relax the muscles and reduce the pain.

To ease your daughter's painful periods, look for over-the-counter products that contain angelica, basil, clary sage, cramp bark, cypress, geranium, marjoram, passionflower, skullcap, wild yam, or yellow dock root. For acute pain, give your daughter five drops of mother-wort tincture every five minutes, but no more than fifty drops total, until the pain is gone.

Chapter 6 includes several herbal and aromatherapy options for girls with painful periods. Try Cramping-Up Tea (page 164) which contains herbs that help relax cramps and help normalize menstruation. A massage with Menstrual Cramp Oil (page 166), Severe Cramp Extract (page 167), or Spasm Massage Oil (page 167) contain essential oils that help relax the body and ease topical pain.

Premenstrual Syndrome (PMS)

About a third to a half of all females experience premenstrual syndrome. Common symptoms are bloating, breast tenderness, constipation, depression, headache, irritability, and a tendency to overeat.

Some easy ways to alleviate PMS are to eat foods rich in calcium and to get a safe amount of sunshine for vitamin D. Vitamin D promotes calcium absorption, which can help stop cramping.

For depression associated with PMS, try twenty drops of mother-wort tincture two to three times per day. Women tell me that moth-erwort gives them the sensation of a weight being lifted from their bodies, or that they feel as if the "veil is being lifted." St. John's wort is also used for depression; give twenty drops of tincture two to three times a day. In addition, look for herbal products that contain some of the following herbs: alfalfa, blue vervain (*Verbena hastata*), chaste berry, dandelion root and leaf, false unicorn root (*Chamaelirium luteum*), oats, red raspberry, stinging nettle, valerian, and yarrow.

To treat that crampy feeling just before the period starts, make a decoction of two parts dried cramp bark, one part dried red raspberry leaf, and one-half part fresh or dried ginger. Your daughter should drink one cup three times a day for one or two days before her period begins. Another helpful formula for cramps is a decoction of two parts dried red raspberry leaf and one part *each* dried alfalfa, dried cramp bark, and dried stinging nettle. Your daughter should drink one cup three times a day on the day her period begins.

Aromatherapy can be effective, especially for girls who feel weepy or emotional just before their periods begin. Combine five drops *each* essential oils of rose and geranium plus ten drops of clary sage essential oil in one-half cup of carrier oil, such as apricot kernel oil. Use as needed as a massage oil or as a perfume on the neck and chest.

For teen girls who become irritable just before their periods begin, combine ten drops *each* essentials oils of bergamot, clary sage, and nutmeg and five drops geranium essential oil in one-half cup of carrier oil. Dab some on a handkerchief and remind your daughter to inhale the aroma when she's feeling snappish. Alternatively, for a refreshing and therapeutic air mist, add the essential oils to one-half cup of water instead of oil. Pour the mixture into a mister. Your daughter can inhale the mist as needed.

Heavy Periods

Heavy bleeding during periods can be caused by hormonal imbalances, disease, improper diet, or general debility. A teenager could become anemic if this continues over the course of a few cycles, or if there is prolonged bleeding. Consult your daughter's doctor or healthcare practitioner.

Products on the market for this problem are mostly tinctures and teas. Look for ones that contain american cranesbill, beth root, cinnamon, lady's mantle, periwinkle, red raspberry leaf, shepherd's purse, yarrow, or yellow dock root.

A massage with Cypress Oil Massage Blend (page 166) or Periwinkle Blend (page 166) can help reduce menstrual flow. Profuse

Menstruation Regulation Blend (pages 166–167) works similarly to regulate and normalize menstruation. IronWomyn (page 165) is an iron-replenishing extract for anemia.

A Word About Depression

Several herbs are used in the treatment of depression. These include cardamom, motherwort, and St. John's wort. If your teen shows signs of depression beyond the usual moody "teenage blues," she may be clinically depressed. Consult a mental health professional before attempting to treat your child's depression with herbal remedies.

Buying, Gathering, and Preparing Herbs

4

After seeing for themselves how well herbals work for their families, many parents want to make their own remedies. If you are ready to delve further into the world of herbal medicine and make your own, you can buy the herbs you need or grow them, either in a full-fledged herb garden or in pots on your balcony or window ledge.

BUYING HERBS

Always buy organically grown herbs. Most large herb companies fumigate their plants because pests could wipe out their entire stock. Many companies also have begun to irradiate their herbs to kill pests. Buying herbs from a distributor who uses overseas suppliers increases your chances of getting irradiated products.

Using chemically free herbs is as important as eating chemically free foods, but not just for our personal health. When we choose organics, we promote sustainable farming and biodiversity, help reduce pollution, protect the soil and water, and make work safer for farmers and farm workers. Think how much better you will feel, not just physically but emotionally, when you nourish your body and your family with clean, honorably produced food. When we make choices that protect our environment, we are also making choices that protect our bodies.

Buying locally supports your neighbors and smaller farms. Shop for organic herbs at your farmers' market. Get to know the people who grow them. When I buy garlic from the farmer down the road, I know I'm getting fresh and potent garlic that will do its job in my remedies.

If you can't buy locally, seek out organic herbs and herbal products at natural-food stores—usually in the bulk section—or from specialty retailers. Research your source. For a list of recommended online and mail-order suppliers, see pages 191–194.

GROWING YOUR OWN

Gardening books may feature elaborate herbal knot gardens that look complicated and intimidating, but the fact is, herbs are easy to grow. And they can be grown just about anywhere there is good soil, sunshine, and water (and maybe a little compost once in a while). You can grow herbs in a small plot in the yard; in a corner of your garden; or in pots on your porch, patio, or kitchen window sill. Basic information about growing herbs can be found in almost any gardening book.

When planting your herb garden, try to plant from seeds as much as possible. This saves money, of course, and it also teaches children about gardening and how things grow. Don't be concerned with straight-as-an-arrow row planting or pulling every last weed. Gardening is supposed to be a fun stress reliever. Just trust in the process and allow yourself to observe the journey from seed to harvest.

WILDCRAFTING

Wildcrafting simply means gathering plants from the wild—from fields, meadows, mountainsides, natural areas, pastures, or anywhere you can legally pick herbs. If you are not on public lands, request permission from the property owner.

You should follow certain rules when wildcrafting, not only for how to pick the herbs but also for respecting nature. Before gathering any herbs, study the environment. Never pick herbs in contaminated habitats, such as areas along highways, beside factories, or near any other structure that may have tainted the earth. Do not pick herbs that are growing where you see dead and dying plants; garbage in the undergrowth, oil-slicked puddles, or sewage. Remember that plants store the environment's energy, water, and air. If the area is polluted, then the herb is most likely polluted as well.

Never harvest more than you can use, and never deplete a local plant stand. I often tell my students not to pick more than 10 percent

Identifying Wild Herb Plants

A good field guide can be your most important tool if you plan to pick herbs in the wild. I recommend the following:

A Field Guide to Medicinal Plants and Herbs: Of Eastern and Central North America by Steven Foster, James A. Duke, and Roger Tory Peterson (A similar version of this Peterson Field Guide covers western medicinal plants and herbs.)

Botany in a Day by Thomas J. Elpel

Field Guide to Medicinal Wild Plants by Bradford Angier

Growing 101 Herbs that Heal: Gardening Techniques, Recipes, and Remedies by Tammi Hartung

Identifying and Harvesting Edible and Medicinal Plants by Steve Brill

Shanleya's Quest: A Botany Adventure for Kids Ages 9–99 by Thomas J. Elpel

Here are some tips for learning how to identify herb plants:

- Always carry a camera and take pictures of plants you don't recognize so you can look them up later.
- Hire a local guide to lead identification walks. Many botanical societies, gardening clubs, boy or girl scout troops, organic gardening associations, nature preserves, forest preserves, natural-food stores, and alternative health clinics can recommend someone.
- Plant herbs yourself and label them with name stakes.

of an existing herbal stand or patch. (However, that percentage can vary depending on the size of the patch.) Other people in the community may also want to harvest the plants. Also consider that animals and insects rely on plants for food, pollination, and other necessities.

Do not pick protected plants. Find out which plants are protected in your area and use a good field guide to identify them. Just because a plant appears to be plentiful does not automatically mean you can pick it. And a plant that is not protected in one area may be protected in another, so find out which plants are protected wherever you wildcraft. If in doubt, don't harvest the plant. Information about protected plants can be found on state wildlife websites (most will have a link to this information) and the USDA website at http://plants.usda.gov/threat.html.

I believe wildcrafting has a spiritual aspect. Native Americans and others who practice nature-based religions ask before taking and always give something back to the earth. Traditionally, indigenous people have used tobacco, cornmeal, or another valued commodity as a special offering. We are all indigenous peoples of the planet, so we should all give back. Think about what you can give back when you take. Planting roots or seeds is a great way to replenish and give back, as is donating to conservation projects.

HARVESTING

An herb's harvest time is best determined by the herb's growth stage rather than by a specific date or month. Most herbs are ready to be harvested just as the flower buds appear. At this stage of growth, the herb's leaves contain the maximum amount of volatile oils, giving the greatest flavor and fragrance to the finished product.

Herbs should be collected in dry weather. If it's been damp all season, let the plants air-dry on a towel before using. Turn them often to help them dry out.

When you want to use fresh herbs, simply pick a few leaves or sprigs here and there as needed throughout the season. If you are harvesting a lot at one time for drying, leave some of the foliage so the plant can continue to grow. Careful pruning ensures new growth. Take no more than 60 percent of the foliage from most annuals at any one harvest. When harvesting short-lived annuals, such as coriander and dill, cut the whole plantar once and then replant for a new crop. Leave about half the foliage on perennials. When harvesting biennial herbs, pick the leaves as needed the first year, but wait until the seeds set the second year to increase your supply of plants. To harvest specific parts of a plant (flowers, roots, and so on), refer to the following guidelines.

Bark

Bark is harvested in both the spring and fall because that's when the sap of the plant is running. In the spring, the sap runs from the roots upward to the parts of the plant that are above ground. The reverse is true in the fall. Bark should easily peel from the wood.

Never cut through bark in a solid line around the trunk; this will kill the tree. It's best to take bark from wood that has already been felled. Harvest bark from broken branches, twigs, and peeling sections. Don't use bark from rotting or dead branches.

Flowers

Flowers usually contain the best medicine the plant has to offer, so harvest them right after they have fully opened. Do not take broken, bruised, or diseased flowers.

Leaves

Leaves should be gathered in their prime. The optimum time to collect leaves is in clear, dry weather, in the morning after the dew is gone and the sun is still low. Leaves have the most volatile oils at this time. Do not harvest leaves that are contaminated, discolored, or diseased. If you're gathering a flowering plant, harvest just before the plant flowers or immediately after full flowering occurs. (During flowering, the plant is giving most of its energy to make beautiful flowers.)

Roots

Roots should be harvested in the fall when the plants are dormant. At any other time of the growing season, the roots are circulating nutrients and energy to feed the plant's foliage. (To remember this, use the herb gatherer's saying: "Nutrients and healing power fall to the root; in spring, they spring to the plant.") Roots hold the plant's lifeblood and should be collected in a manner that honors this. When digging roots, try to leave some of the root for replanting so the plant can continue to grow and produce.

To harvest roots you will need a strong shovel or trowel and a container to put the roots in. I like to use a light canvas bag because the texture removes a substantial amount of surface dirt from the roots. A box or paper bag also works fine. While the roots are still in the bag, remove as much dirt from them as you can, then pour out the excess dirt. You can wear a pair of canvas gloves and rub the roots with your hands to achieve the same effect.

When you get home, use a vegetable brush under running water to wash off as much of the remaining dirt as you can, as quickly as you can, so the root won't absorb water and become soft. Let the

Harvesting Annuals, Biennials, and Perennials

Annuals, such as basil, complete their growth in one season. Trim them during the growing season any time you need a few leaves. Use a sharp knife, scissors, or pruning shears to cut just above a leaf or a pair of leaves, allowing four to six inches of the stem to remain for later growth. (Do not harvest leaves from plants that you are growing for seed. Allow the plants to mature fully before harvesting the seed and the leaves.) In the fall, annuals can be cut back quite severely—if not uprooted and removed from the garden completely—since they will not regenerate or grow back unless reseeded.

Perennials, such as delphinium and lavender, die back on their own and produce new growth the next season. Most perennial herbs will be ready to harvest just prior to or during the early part of July, with a second harvest possible in September in most parts of the United States. Only about one-third of the top growth should be removed at a time. In some cases, only the leafy tips should be removed. At the end of the growing season, cut them about halfway down.

Biennials, such as anise, parsley, and parsnips, require two growing seasons to go from seed to seed. They may reseed themselves if they are organic and not genetically modified. Consider them short-term perennials. Leaves may be harvested the first year, but I think it is better to wait until the plant is in its second year. At the end of the growing season, cut biennials about halfway down.

root dry completely. Using a fresh, oil-based wet root will cause your remedies to spoil.

Seeds

Seeds should be harvested in their prime. This isn't always easy because they tend to fall off or float away in the breeze when they're ready. To harvest seeds, collect the seed heads when they are turning brown by cutting them off the plants. Dry them on a screen or a tray made of very fine wire mesh. Store them in a covered jar or tin in a cool, dark, and dry spot until needed. So that they will germinate when planted in the spring, some herb seeds have to be frozen in advance. Be sure to find out if this is true for the seed you're collecting. Obviously, this is only important if you plan to plant the seed.

PRESERVING HERBS

Preserving fresh herbs guarantees that you'll have a supply to carry you through the season. If you want to store your herbs for more than a few days, you can either dry them or freeze them. Air-drying is the traditional method, oven drying and freezing are quicker, and microwave drying is handy for small batches. Remove all damaged, discolored, or diseased leaves before trying one of the following methods.

Drying

For medicinal uses, dried herbs are usually preferable to fresh ones, because they contain more concentrated amounts of the herb's active ingredients. Dried herbs are easy to store and keep exceedingly well, so you'll always have herbs readily available.

There are many ways to dry herbs, from elaborate screening trays in a greenhouse to gas or electric ovens in an urban kitchen. The important thing to remember is that no matter how you dry herbs— whether you hang them from the barn rafters or zap them in your microwave—the point is to dry them, not cook them.

Most herbs can be dried, but there are exceptions. Garlic and stinging nettle should always be used fresh or frozen because their active compounds deteriorate when they are dried. Also, use freshly picked echinacea plants instead of dried.

When drying whole branches or stems, strip off the flowers, smaller leaves, and very small stems. Wash the branches or stems under cool water and gently pat them dry with a dish towel or paper towel. Gather five to eight stems together and tie them into a bundle with twine or kitchen string. Place the bundle in a brown paper bag with the stems extending out of the open end and tie the bag closed around the stems. Hang the bag in a dark, warm place (70 to 80 degrees Fahrenheit). Depending on the temperature and humidity, drying time will take two to four weeks.

Air-Drying

Air-drying is a time-honored technique for preserving herbs. Leafy herbs are usually hung upside down to dry. Gather fresh herbs in a small bunch of three to five stems *each* for large, leafy herbs, such as sage, or six to eight stems *each* for smaller herbs, such as thyme. Secure the stem end of each bundle with a rubber band. To dry seeds, hang the seed heads on their stalks upside down in a paper bag. The seeds will fall into the bag as they dry. Most herbs will dry to the touch in one to three days depending on the amount of humidity in the air.

Dehydrating

You can use a food dehydrator to dry herbs. I recommend the Nesco-American Harvest and Excalibur dehydrators. You can also get good-quality dehydrators from businesses that cater to the raw-food community. Follow the manufacturer's instructions.

Oven Drying

A conventional gas or electric oven, or even a microwave oven, can be used to dry herbs quickly. This must be done carefully, though, because drying herbs too quickly at too high a temperature results in the loss of flavor, oils, and color.

To dry herbs in an electric oven, preheat the oven to 100 degrees Fahrenheit. In a gas oven, the heat from the pilot light is ideal for drying herbs; there's no need to turn on the oven. Place leaves and stems on a cookie sheet or in a shallow pan and dry them in the oven for three to four hours with the oven door open.

Roots take longer to dry because of their thickness. Roots that can be dried successfully include burdock, comfrey, ginger, ginseng, and sassafras. To dry roots, scrub them clean with a brush. Slice larger roots in half lengthwise; smaller roots may be left whole. Preheat the oven to about 175 degrees Fahrenheit. Place the roots in a shallow pan and dry them in the oven for three to four hours with the oven door cracked.

Microwave/Drying

In a microwave-safe dish, lay out clean stems or leaves evenly on paper towels. Place another layer of paper towels on top of the herbs. Microwave on high for one to three minutes, turning the stems or stirring the leaves every thirty seconds. Keep a close eye on the drying herbs and stop the microwave if you see any signs of smoke or charring. If this happens, try a new batch for a shorter period of time. When you determine the right drying time, jot it down for future reference.

Some herbs, especially those with flowers and flower petals, maintain extremely good color, form, and flavor when dried in the microwave. Others, though, seem to cook and become crispy but flavorless. Experiment to see which herbs dry best.

I do not advocate the microwave method. I think microwaves disturb the herb's energy, but that is just my opinion. Ultimately, we all have to do whatever works for our lifestyles and families.

Salt Drying

Herbs can also be dried in salt. Salt draws moisture from the herbs and absorbs some of their essential oils. You can use the flavored salt to season your food. To make herbed seasoning salt to sprinkle on foods, wash, dry, and mince the leaves of the herbs you want to use. To preserve sprigs to crumble into foods, wash and dry sprigs of the herbs you want to use, then remove and discard any thick stems or inedible parts.

Salt drying works best with thin-leaved herbs, such as dill, marjoram, rosemary, savory, tarragon, and thyme. You can also dry thicker herbs in salt—just use fewer leaves and more salt. To dry herbs with salt, pour a ¼-inch deep layer of kosher salt, sea salt, or another noniodized salt into a container with a tight-fitting lid, such as a canning jar or freezer container. Sprinkle the minced herbs over the salt layer. If you are using sprigs, place them on top of the salt layer. Cover the herbs with another ¼-inch layer of salt. Continue layering the herbs and salt until you've used up all the herbs. End with a layer of salt. Cover or seal tightly.

The herbs will dry in about a week. To make seasoning salt, mix the salt and herbs together well, then pour the mixture into a small, airtight container to keep on your kitchen counter or table. To use the dried sprigs, simply pull out individual sprigs, brush off the salt, and crumble the herbs into food.

Tray Drying

Tray drying is usually used for short-stemmed herbs, such as thyme, or for individual leaves, such as basil. You can use an old window screen or make your own small drying tray with 2 by 2-inch lumber and a piece of cloth or screen. Wash and dry the herbs you want to dry, then lay them out on the drying tray. Keep the tray in a warm, dark place until the herbs are dry. Leaves will require a couple of days to a week to dry; flowers, about two weeks; and thinly sliced roots, up to a month. The time it takes for an herb to dry thoroughly will depend on the type of herb, the humidity, and the temperature.

Freezing

Freezing is a quick and easy way to preserve many herbs. It's especially good for herbs that tend to lose their flavor when dried, such as basil, chives, french tarragon, lovage, and parsley. When the frozen herbs are thawed, however, they are limp and not especially attractive, so they're best used in teas, tinctures, and syrups.

To prepare leaves for freezing, chop them and place them in plastic containers or bags. Another method is to purée herbs in a blender with a little water or olive oil and freeze the purée in ice cube trays. When the easy-to-use cubes are ready, remove them from the trays and store them in plastic containers or bags in the freezer. Label all frozen herbs with their names and date of storage, and use them within six months.

Making Candy

American colonists couldn't run to the store to buy candy when they had a sweet tooth, so they made their own sweet treats out of herbs. They candied young angelica stems and ginger, preserving the herb and bringing out its flavor with a crystal-sugar shell. Although their sweets may not replace modern candies, they are wonderful as dessert garnishes or edible decorations on cakes and pastries.

Cookbooks from the 1700s recommended the following process for candied angelica: Cook young angelica stems in boiling water until tender. Peel off and discard the fibrous strings. Return the stems to simmering water, and cook until they turn very green. Remove the stems from the water, and let them dry.

Place the dried, cooked stems in a bowl or on a tray. Cover the stems with an equal amount of superfine granulated white sugar (one pound of sugar per one pound of stems). Let stand for two days. Place the mixture in a large saucepan and boil until the sugar melts into clear syrup. Drain off the syrup. Cover with an equal amount of sugar (again, one pound of sugar per one pound of stems). Remove the stems from the sugar and place on plates to dry in a warm place.

Violets and rose petals are even easier to candy: Brush a little egg white all over each flower and dip it in superfine or powdered sugar. Let dry. Store in an airtight container.

Making Syrup

Sugar syrups flavored with herbs can add taste to cold drinks and baked foods, such as custards. To make herb-flavored sugar syrup, simmer two parts water and one part sugar in a saucepan. Add a handful of fresh herbs, stems and all, to the simmering syrup. Cook until the herbs lose color and the syrup is aromatic, about fifteen to thirty minutes. Use the syrup immediately, or cool and store the syrup in covered jars in the refrigerator.

STORING HERBS

Store your dried herbs in sterilized, dark glass containers with airtight lids. Label the container with the name of the herb, including its Latin genus and species name, and the date. (Labeling is very important. Many dried herbs look and smell alike, making it easy to use the wrong herb, which could be dangerous.) Store dried herbs at room temperature in a cool, dry place away from sunlight, moisture, children, and pets.

Another storage method is to place the herbs in labeled freezer bags and keep them in the freezer for up to six months. You can also store herbs in brown paper bags, which must be kept dry and away from light to prevent bleaching. To keep bugs away, place the paper bags inside plastic containers.

Because moisture can cause herbs to mold, make sure herbs are completely dry before they are stored. If you open a container of stored herbs and find mold, discard the herbs. Do not use moldy herbs.

Dried herbs, except for a few types of roots, have a relatively short lifespan. Dried flowers, leaves, roots, and other herb parts keep for about one year when stored at or just below room temperature. Chinese medicine uses very old roots; however, in Western herbalism, herbs generally do not have a long shelf life. If you've dried more herbs than you're going to use, consider freezing them. Wrap them in freezer paper, and place the paper packet in a zippered plastic freezer bag or a plastic freezer container.

Making Your Own Herbal Remedies

5

These days, prepared herbal remedies are sold almost everywhere, including natural-food stores, supermarkets, pharmacies, and big-box discount stores. You can find the usual teas and capsules alongside specialty products for particular conditions, such as teas formulated for sore throats or oils for ear infections.

Instead of buying herbal remedies, you may want to try your hand at making your own. Most homemade herbal remedies are made in the form of decoctions, extracts, infusions, and tinctures. You can also make compresses, liniments, poultices, salves, and more.

HERB QUALITY

How can you judge the quality of an herb? Whether you grow your own, purchase from a natural-food store, harvest from the wild, or buy from a bulk supplier, consider the following when judging whether an herb will be effective:

- Fresh herbs should retain their fresh color, aroma, and taste. Their leaves and roots should look alive and healthy.
- Dried herbs should remain pretty much in their whole state. The flowers should look like flowers, the leaves like leaves, and so on.
- Dried herbs should not be mostly stems and "dust." The more broken down the herb, the shorter its shelf life. Sift through the dried herb with your fingers, and look at the color and texture.
- Dried herbs should smell and taste vibrant and fresh, not musty and old.

The ultimate test for any herb is to use it in a remedy and gauge its potency and effectiveness. This is also the best way to evaluate whether or not to purchase from a particular supplier in the future.

EQUIPMENT

Once you have your herbs, gather together the equipment you'll need to make your remedies. This includes pots and pans of various sizes, including a 6-quart pot and a stock pot. Stainless steel, copper, or enamel-coated pans are best. Do not use aluminum, Teflon-coated, or other types of coated cookware. Because herbal medicines are often served as teas, you'll also need high-quality china tea pots that can withstand boiling water and a lot of use. Use a cup strainer when pouring the tea.

Following is a list of additional equipment you might need. None of this has to be fancy. You probably have most of these in your kitchen already:

- bottles and jars, glass (reuse baby-food, canning, and small condiment jars, or buy new jars for this purpose)
- canning jars and lids
- cheesecloth or muslin
- cookie sheets, two uncoated, heavy gauge (adjust baking time for insulated sheets)
- double boiler
- droppers or pipettes
- french press coffeepot (can be used instead of a teapot or to strain tinctures)
- funnels, metal, two or three in different sizes
- jars, plastic, 2- to 4-ounce double-walled, insulated, with lids
- measuring cups, glass
- measuring spoons, stainless steel
- muslin bags, 8- and 12-inch
- orifice reducers (to adjust the size of jar openings)
- salve pots, 2- to 4-ounce glass, and lids

- screening material or window screens for drying herbs
- spray bottles
- strainers, all types, including tea strainers

DECOCTIONS

A decoction is the concentrated liquor that remains after heating or boiling down an herb, specifically, the more tenacious plant parts, such as the bark, nuts, or roots. I really like to let my decoctions steep for a generous amount of time—a few hours sometimes—because I suggest teas for so many tonic and medicinal uses.

Decoctions are used to make teas and are ingredients in such things as compresses, liniments, and hair rinses. To make a decoction, simmer one to two tablespoons of the herb in one cup of water for twenty minutes. Steep for twenty to thirty minutes. Strain the decoction into a dry jar and screw on the lid tightly. Store decoctions in the refrigerator or a cool place. Decoctions don't keep well, so plan to use them within forty-eight hours of preparation.

HINT: One way to make decoctions more palatable or desirable to young children is to freeze them into popsicles. Use half decoction and half fruit juice in each mold.

INFUSIONS

An infusion is a remedy made by soaking plant parts or dried herbs in a liquid. Herbal tea is the most well-known and popular herbal infusion. The general formula for making herbal tea is to use about one teaspoon of dried herb per one cup of boiling water. Steep the tea for ten to twenty minutes, strain the tea, and discard the herbs. Stored properly in the refrigerator, tea infusions can last one or two days.

An infused oil is a popular and easy medium for administering an herb's healing compounds. Infused oils are simple to make. Merely place the fresh or dried herb in a clean or sterilized jar and cover it with oil, preferably olive oil, although sunflower oil and grapeseed oil can also be used if you have those on hand. Some herbalists follow formulas and ratios of herbs to oil, but I usually just pack the jar with as much fresh herb as will fit and cover it completely with oil. As a result, my oils come out richly colored. For example, St. John's wort oil is bright red, lavender oil is purple, and plantain and comfrey oils are spring green.

Once the herbs and oil are in the jar, there are a couple of ways to steep an infusion. One method is to place the jar in the sunshine during the day for two weeks, then strain the oil through a piece of cheesecloth. (For a really potent oil, repeat the process, reusing the infused oil in a jar full of fresh herbs.) Strain the infusion through a piece of cheesecloth into a clean, dry jar. Screw on the lid, and store the jar in a dry, cool place. This method is particularly good when you are making colorful oils with herbs such as rose hips and St. John's wort because the long steep time extracts more bioflavonoids and active constituents.

A second method is to place the jar containing the herbs and oil in simmering water in a slow cooker. The water level should be about one inch below the jar's lid. Keep an eye on the water level and don't let it go down. Maintain it by refilling with boiling water as needed. After four hours, remove the jar from the slow cooker. When the jar is cool enough to handle, strain the infused oil through a piece of cheesecloth into a clean, dry jar. Screw on the lid and store the jar in a dry, cool place.

You can also use a double boiler to make an infusion. Place the herbs in the top of the double boiler until it is one-half to three-quarters full. Cover the herbs with the vegetable oil of your choice, and place the mixture over gently simmering water for about three hours. Remove the mixture from the heat and allow it to cool. Strain the mixture through a piece of cheesecloth or muslin into clean jars, then discard the herbs and cover the oil tightly.

For some additional, extra-strong energy, place infused oils under the light of a full moon for one night. Infused oils will keep up to two years. Discard if mold forms.

EXTRACTS

An extract is a remedy that contains the active ingredient(s) of an herb in a concentrated form. These are usually extracted by soaking the herb for a long period in alcohol or pure vegetable glycerin. Glycerin is recommended for children's remedies because it is sweet and helps the medicine go down. (If using glycerin, use dried, not fresh, herbs.)

To make an extract, place fresh or dried herb in a clean, dry jar. Add enough liquid so that the level is three fingers higher than the dried herb or two fingers higher than the fresh herb. Cover the jar and allow it to sit in the sunlight for a few days. For extra potency, place the jar under a full moon all night or in the sun all afternoon. Store the jar in a cupboard or other dark place. After two weeks, the extract will be saturated with color from the herbs. Strain it through a piece of cheesecloth and press as much liquid as you can from the herb before discarding. The extract is now ready to use.

Always store extracts in a dry, dark place. Alcohol extracts last two to five years; glycerin extracts last one to three years.

Among herbalists, it is a time-honored tradition to begin making extracts on the eve of the new moon and strain on the full moon. The waxing powers of the moon extract the greatest amount of therapeutic agents from the herbs.

TINCTURES

Tinctures and extracts are made by extracting the active properties of the herb in alcohol. A tincture is traditionally a diluted extract. Unfortunately, the terms "extract" and "tincture" are often interchanged and misused these days. Most extracts are 40 percent alcohol, whereas tinctures may have the same alcohol content but not as much of the herb. When purchasing tinctures, read the label carefully to make sure you are buying what you think you are buying.

Commercial tinctures and extracts are labeled with the recommended dosage, usually ten to thirty drops, three times per day. However, tincture dosages are best determined individually based on the severity of the illness and the strength of the herb. To determine the correct dose, follow my recipes, consult a professional herbalist, or rely on a couple of good reference books.

Making tinctures is actually pretty simple. However, if you want the variety that most parents need in a well-stocked medicine chest, it's probably cheaper to buy tinctures.

To make a tincture, you will need dried or fresh herbs; 80- to 100-proof vodka, brandy, or rum; labels and markers; wide-mouthed glass mason jars with lids (the size depends on how much tincture you want to make); and unbleached cheesecloth or muslin.

Place the herb in the jar. I usually fill a quart jar two inches from the top. Completely cover the herb with the vodka, brandy, or rum. When using dried herbs, a good ratio to follow is about one part herb to five parts alcohol. With fresh herbs, use one part herb to three parts alcohol. Add one more inch of alcohol if you're using fresh herbs, and two more inches if you're using dried. (Dried herbs absorb more liquid and expand.) Close the jar tightly, and place it in a dark place, such as a cabinet or closet.

Shake the jar gently every day. The extract will be ready to decant in four to eight weeks. Strain the liquid through a piece of cheesecloth or muslin into another jar or a dark-colored tincture bottle. Squeeze or press the soaked herbs, extracting as much of the remaining liquid as you can. Close the bottle, and label it with the name of the herb and the date. Tinctures will keep several months to several years when stored in dark glass bottles in a cool place away from sunlight.

ESSENTIAL OILS

Essential oils are highly aromatic healing substances distilled from plants. They are, simply, the oils of the plant and contain the true essence of the herb—its highly concentrated, potent, and volatile aromatic compounds. Essential oils are an intense form of plant remedy and aromatherapy. A little goes a long, long way. The chemical properties of the oils (which, interestingly enough, are not all that oily) can be balancing, cleansing, deodorizing, or toning. Essential oils can be used to treat children, with some caveats. (See Essential Caveats, below).

Store essential oils in dark glass bottles in a cool, dark place. Seal the bottles tightly with nonrubber lids to prevent evaporation. Essential oils should be used within a year or, if mixed with carrier oil, within three months.

Essential Caveats

Although essential oils are healing and add an aesthetic dimension to therapies such as baths, massages, and steams, they should be used with knowledge and care. Almost all essential oils should be diluted. (Refer to the individual recipe for the remedy.) Do not apply essential oils directly to the skin. Never give them internally unless a professional herbalist or medical practitioner prescribes them. Do not allow essential oils to touch the eyes, mouth, and other tender, mucous membranes. In addition, keep essential oils away from flames and store them out of the reach of children and pets. The following lists outline special cautions.

Always Dilute These Essential Oils

The following essential oils should always be diluted with carrier oil, such as apricot kernel oil or olive oil:

- anise
- bergamot
  (use only five drops to four tablespoons of carrier oil)
- clove bud
- coriander
- eucalyptus blue gum
- fennel
- hyssop
- nutmeg
- parsley seed
- spanish sage
- tagetes
  (use only five drops to four tablespoons of carrier oil)
- tea tree
- thyme
- verbena
- west indian bay
- white camphor

Avoid These Essential Oils

The following essential oils are dangerous and should *never* be used to treat babies and children:

- benzoin
- boldo
- calamus
- mugwort
- mustard
- pennyroyal
- rue
- sassafras
- tansy
- wormseed

Known Irritants

The following essential oils are known irritants. They should be used very carefully and be highly diluted (5 percent of a blend with carrier oil):

- anise
- basil
- black pepper
- cajeput
- cinnamon
- clove bud
- lemongrass
- lemon
- parsley seed
- peppermint
- pine needle
- thyme
- virginian cedarwood
- white camphor

Avoid in Sunshine

The following essential oils can make skin sensitive to sunlight. Don't use them topically on a child who is going to be exposed to sunshine:

- angelica root
- bergamot
- bitter orange
- grapefruit
- lemon
- lime
- sweet orange
- tangerine

Special Considerations

Be aware of essential oils that have dangerous side effects or should not be used to treat children with specific health concerns.

- Avoid essential oils of boldo, calamus, and sassafras; they've been shown to be carcinogenic.
- If your child has epilepsy, do not use essential oils of fennel, hyssop, rosemary, or spanish sage.
- If your child has hypoglycemia, avoid essential oil of geranium.
- If your child has kidney problems, avoid essential oils of coriander, juniper, and sandalwood, unless prescribed by a professional herbalist or medical practitioner.

Aromatherapy

Essential oils are used therapeutically in the healing practice of aromatherapy. They can be diffused into the environment, inhaled directly, or applied topically. Our bodies use the aromatic molecules of essential oils both for healing and peace of mind.

Aromatherapy works because our olfactory system is connected to points in the brain called the limbic system, where our most instinctive feelings and sexual emotions reside. Smell is a powerful sense that can evoke memories, feelings, and attachments. When stimulated by smell, the limbic system releases chemicals that affect the central nervous system.

A good aromatherapist will know and understand the subtle differences among essential oils and how their chemical constituents affect a child's body. Parents can use simple aromatherapy remedies to make a child feel better, such as spritzing a room spray, adding a few drops of essential oil to bath water or massage oil, or putting a drop of essential oil on a cloth and tucking it under a pillow. Such noninvasive remedies create very little stress or resistance.

Almost all essential oils should be diluted with a carrier oil, such as almond, jojoba, or even olive oil, before being applied to the skin so they don't irritate. The essential oils of lavender and tea tree are generally considered safe for teens and adults for direct skin application; however, for babies and children, I always recommend that they also be diluted.

When using essential oils with babies or children, always reduce the recommended amount on the package or bottle by half or more. An infant should be prescribed no more than one or two drops; older children may have up to one-quarter of the adult dose. When in doubt, use infused herbal oils instead of essential oils for infants. For most applications, use one drop of essential oil per five milliliters or one teaspoon of carrier oil. In a bathtub of water, use no more than five to ten drops.

Children usually have more sensitive skin than adults. If your child's skin is extra sensitive, apply a very small amount of diluted oil on the inside of his arm and wait one hour. If irritation develops, rub the area well with pure carrier oil and wash it with soap and water. Dilute the oil even more, and try again.

LINIMENTS

A liniment is an herbal extraction in a liquid, such as alcohol, oil, or vinegar, which is rubbed into the skin to treat arthritis, inflammations, sore muscles, and strains. To make one of my favorite

liniments, place four ounces *each* fresh or dried peppermint and eucalyptus leaves in a 16-ounce jar. Cover with a pint of vodka or vinegar.
(Do not use rubbing alcohol.) Let the mixture sit in a dry place for
fourteen days and shake the contents twice a day. (You can also add a
few drops of essential oil, such as eucalyptus, peppermint, or rosemary,
if you like.) For an "instant" liniment, mix one teaspoon of essential oil
of peppermint, eucalyptus, or rosemary with one-half cup of vodka.

SALVES

When my boys were small, I was never without lavender essential oil, peppermint tincture, and Soothing Salve (page 175).
With just these three remedies, I was able to manage most issues
that came up when I was out hiking for the day with my children.
Salves are the primary tool in my medicine chest. Most of my family's aches and pains, bruises, cuts, scrapes, and strains are treated
with salves.

Salves are creams or emollients that provide barrier protection
while carrying medicinal benefits. When buying prepared herbal
salves, look for the appropriate herb, of course, but also make sure
the remaining ingredients are ones you recognize and have names you
can understand.

Making your own salve may sound laborious, but it's done simply
by melting grated beeswax with oil in a double boiler, stirring in the
herbs or essential oils, pouring the mixture into containers, and allowing it to solidify. If the salve is too hard, melt it and add more oil;
if it's too soft, melt it and add more grated beeswax.

In addition to the herbs and essential oils, you will need an oil
such as almond, apricot kernel, grapeseed, or olive; beeswax or vegan
wax, such as candelilla wax or coconut oil; a pan in which to melt
the wax and mix the ingredients; and containers, such as glass salve
pots and mason jars, in which to store the salve. (See Suppliers, pages
191–194, for sources for beeswax, hard oils for vegan salves, liquid
oils, essential oils, and containers.)

If you'd like to try your hand at making salves, start out with
some basic ones that can be used for many common conditions.
Calendula salve, for example, is gentle and versatile; it is excellent
for eczema, diaper rash, and dry, cracked skin. Comfrey salve cools
down inflamed skin and helps heal rashes and other skin problems.

(Caution: Comfrey should only be used externally. See page 60.) Plantain salve has strongly astringent and soothing properties and helps to reduce the pain of wounds, stings, and insect bites. In addition, it helps to stop bleeding.

COMPRESSES

A compress is made by soaking a piece of cloth in a hot decoction or infusion and applying it as hot as can be tolerated to the affected area. When the compress has cooled, soak it again in the hot decoction or infusion and reapply until there is some relief.

Cold compresses are useful for small bruises and other minor boo-boos. Soak the compress in cold water that is mixed with the desired herb. When my family is on the go and I need to make a compress quickly, I soak it in extracts, sometimes diluted in water and sometimes straight, depending on the strength needed.

A different type of compress is called a *fomentation*, which is an especially good treatment for colds, flu, pain, and swelling. Soak a soft cloth, such as a cloth diaper or washcloth, in the desired hot tea infusion. Squeeze out some of the excess liquid; the cloth should be very wet but not dripping. Apply the cloth as hot as can be tolerated. To hold in the heat, cover the cloth with a warm piece of flannel or another cloth or towel. Repeat as needed. (Microwave ovens are great for heating cloth. Electric or gas ovens that are set on low heat can work as well.)

POULTICES

A poultice is similar to a compress except that fresh plant parts are used instead of decoctions or infusions. Poultices are considered more "active" than compresses. They are used to stimulate circulation, ease aches and pains, or draw impurities from the body through the skin; therefore, they need to remain in place for a few hours at a time.

There are several ways to make a poultice. The simplest method is to mash or crush the fresh plant with a rolling pin on a clean cloth, and fold up the cloth so the plant material is wrapped inside. Place the poultice on the affected area and wrap it with another cloth to hold in body heat.

For a steamed poultice, mash the plant with a mortar and pestle or run it through a food processor. Heat this pulp in a colander over boiling water or in a steamer, or mix it with a small amount of boiling water. Remove it from the heat, and let sit until it is still very warm but cool enough to handle (about ten minutes). Apply the mushy plant pulp directly to the skin as hot as can be tolerated, holding it in place with a gauze bandage. As soon as the poultice cools, apply another poultice. A hot water bottle can be held against the bandage to keep the poultice warm.

To make a steamed poultice quickly, simmer enough herbs to cover the affected area in water for two minutes. Drain off the water and squeeze out the excess liquid. Rub a little vegetable oil into the affected area to prevent the poultice from sticking, and apply the warm herbs to the skin. Bandage the herbs in place using strips of gauze or cotton fabric, and leave in place two to three hours. Wrapping the poultice in wool cloth will keep it warm longer. Change the poultice when it cools.

PLASTERS

A plaster is similar to a poultice, but dried herbs are typically used. Grind the dried herbs into a powder using a blender, food processor, coffee grinder, or mortar and pestle. Make a paste by mixing one tablespoon of the powdered herb with a little boiling water or hot apple cider vinegar. Smear the herb paste on a piece of wool or gauze, cover it with another piece of wool or gauze, and apply this herb paste "sandwich" or plaster to the skin. If you're using fresh herbs for plasters, pulverize them in a food processor or a blender, or finely chop or mash them by hand.

Plasters are helpful for treating general aches and pains, arthritis, back pain, chronic injuries, frozen shoulders, muscle pains and strains, tennis elbow, and sciatica. They should not be used on open wounds, damaged skin, or irritated skin. And they should not be used on children age two and younger.

Depending on the herbs used, plasters can be left in place for several hours, even overnight. Reduce this time, however, when using herbs that could irritate the skin, such as garlic or horseradish.

LOZENGES

Lozenges, or pastilles, are easy-to-make, portable herbal preparations, mainly used to help aid digestion, alleviate sore throats,
calm coughs, and freshen breath.

To make lozenges, mix powdered herbs together in a large bowl.
Add a small amount of honey and a little water and stir. Keep stirring,
adding water a little at a time until the mixture reaches a doughlike
consistency. It will be sticky because of the honey.

With your hands, roll the dough into balls or disks about ½ to ¾
inch in diameter. Roll the balls in ground carob or slippery elm, then
place them on cookie sheets. Set them on the kitchen counter if it's a
warm, dry day, or place them in the oven at the lowest temperature
setting (in a gas oven, heat from the pilot light will be sufficient). Dry
the lozenges completely (this will take thirty to sixty minutes) and let
them cool completely.

SYRUPS

Many prepared herb-based syrups are available at health-food
stores. Instructions for their use and storage are provided on
the label. A homemade herbal syrup should keep up to one month in
the refrigerator. However, if it contains glycerin or alcohol, it will last
up to six months. Discard syrups if mold appears.

Easy Recipes for Homemade Remedies

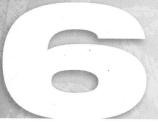

Dozens of herbal products can be found in supermarkets, natural-food stores, and drugstores, but making remedies at home can be less expensive and more fulfilling. This chapter provides recipes for homemade remedies to treat many common childhood illnesses and health conditions.

Equivalents

60 drops	= 1 teaspoon
1 teaspoon	= 4 milliliters
1 ounce (dry)	= 28.4 grams
1 fluid ounce	= 2 tablespoons or 29.57 milliliters
1 teaspoon tincture	= 2 "00" capsules

Acne Blemish Remover Formula YIELD: ABOUT 1 CUP

2 teaspoons dried dandelion root

2 teaspoons dried red clover flowers

1 teaspoon dried alfalfa leaves

1 teaspoon dried echinacea flowers

½ teaspoon cayenne

1 cup boiling water

Add the dandelion root, red clover flowers, alfalfa leaves, echinacea flowers, and cayenne to the boiling water. Steep for 20 minutes. Strain the liquid into a container and discard the herbs. Apply the liquid to the affected area with a cotton swab. Stored in a sealed glass jar in the refrigerator, Acne Blemish Remover Formula will keep for 48 hours.

Acne Poultice YIELD: 1 POULTICE

1 teaspoon ground chaparral

1 teaspoon dried dandelion root

1 teaspoon dried yellow dock root

Ground flaxseeds (optional)

Cornmeal (optional)

Combine the chaparral, dandelion root, and yellow dock root in a small bowl. Add enough water to form a thick paste. If using granulated herbs, add a small amount of ground flaxseeds or cornmeal. Spread the paste ¼-inch thick onto a piece of white cotton. Apply to the affected area and place a towel over the poultice to prevent heat loss.

Acne Toner YIELD: ABOUT 3 CUPS

2 tablespoons dried peppermint leaves

2 tablespoons dried lavender flowers

2 tablespoons dried witch hazel leaves

2½ cups vodka

Combine the peppermint leaves, lavender flowers, and witch hazel leaves with the vodka in a glass container with a lid. Mix well. Cover. Macerate in the refrigerator for 2 weeks. Strain into a bottle and discard the herbs. Cleanse the face daily with a cotton ball or soft cloth dipped in the toner. Stored in a sealed dark-glass bottle and kept in a cool, dark place, Acne Toner will keep for 2 years. Keep out of direct sunlight.

Clear Skin Extract Blend   YIELD: VARIES WITH QUANTITY MADE

1 part cleavers extract

1 part echinacea extract

1 part red clover extract

1 part stinging nettle extract

Combine the extracts in a small bottle. Give 1 teaspoon a day for 6 days. Do not administer on the seventh day. Resume the remedy for another 6 days. If after 1 month of treatment there is no noticeable improvement, consider a different treatment. Stored in a sealed dark-glass bottle and kept in a cool, dark place, Clear Skin Extract Blend will keep for 2 years. Keep out of direct sunlight.

Easy-Does-It Scrub   YIELD: VARIES WITH QUANTITY MADE

1 part rolled oats

1 part salt

1 part almond, avocado, or olive oil

2 to 5 drops chamomile, lavender, patchouli, or tea tree essential oil

Liquid soap

Mix equal parts of rolled oats, salt, and almond oil in a bowl. Add 2 to 5 drops of essential oil (lavender and chamomile are soothing; patchouli and tea tree fight bacteria) and a little liquid soap. Stored in an airtight container, Easy-Does-It Scrub will keep for 2 weeks at room temperature or 2 to 3 months in the refrigerator. To use, rinse the face with water and use the scrub to lather up as usual. Rinse well and pat dry.

Goddess Face Scrub

YIELD: ABOUT 2 CUPS

1 cup finely ground dried chamomile flowers

¼ cup ground dried elder flowers

¼ ground rolled oats

1 teaspoon honey

1 teaspoon dried red clover flowers

1 teaspoon sea salt

Green tea or water

Combine the chamomile flowers, elder flowers, oats, honey, red clover flowers, and salt in a medium bowl. Mix well. Stored in an airtight container, Goddess Face Scrub will keep for 2 weeks at room temperature or 2 to 3 months in the refrigerator. To use, add enough green tea or water to make a paste the consistency of mud and gently scrub the face and neck. Rinse and pat dry. Follow with a gentle toner.

Lavender–Vinegar Lotion

YIELD: ABOUT 4 CUPS

½ cup apple cider vinegar

1 ounce fresh lavender flowers

1 ounce fresh rosemary flowers

Combine all the ingredients in a small glass jar. Cover and steep for 20 days. Strain and discard the herbs. Dilute with 3 cups of water. Stored in an airtight container, Lavender-Vinegar Lotion will keep for 1 to 2 months at room temperature or 2 to 6 months in the refrigerator. Apply to the affected area as needed.

Muddy Mask

YIELD: ABOUT ½ CUP

½ cup cosmetic-grade white or green clay

3 to 4 drops Acne Toner (page 130)

3 to 4 drops echinacea extract

3 to 4 drops ginger extract

1 to 2 drops tea tree essential oil

Make a fine paste by combining all the ingredients in a small bowl. Mix well. Apply liberally to the face. Let dry for a few minutes before removing with a washcloth and warm water. Use Acne Toner (page 130) immediately after to firm and revitalize skin.

Rockin' Rose Toner

YIELD: ABOUT 1 CUP

1 cup witch hazel tincture or commercial witch hazel

2 teaspoons dried rose petals

1 teaspoon dried aloe vera

1 teaspoon dried calendula flowers

1 teaspoon dried chamomile flowers

1 teaspoon dried comfrey leaves

1 teaspoon dried rose hips

1 teaspoon dried yarrow

Combine all the ingredients in a jar. Cover and macerate at room temperature for 2 days. Shake the contents daily. After 2 days, strain into a bottle and discard the rose petals and herbs. Use twice a day on clean skin, applying with a cotton pad, cotton ball, or washcloth. Saturate the cotton and pat the toner gently over the face and neck area and behind the ears. Stored in a sealed dark-glass bottle and kept in a cool, dark place, Rockin' Rose Toner will keep for 2 years. Keep out of direct sunlight.

Witch Hazel–Vodka Conditioning Facial Toner

YIELD: ABOUT ¾ CUP

¼ cup unpeeled cucumber, chopped

¼ cup vodka

¼ cup witch hazel tincture or commercial witch hazel

1 tablespoon olive oil

1 teaspoon almond oil

⅛ teaspoon gentle essential oil, such as geranium, lavender, or rose

Put all the ingredients in a blender. Process on low speed for 30 seconds. Pour into a glass bottle and cap tightly to store. Apply to dry skin with a cotton ball, shaking well before every application. Stored in a sealed dark-glass bottle and kept in a cool, dark place, Witch Hazel–Vodka Conditioning Facial Toner will keep for 2 years. Keep out of direct sunlight.

Zit Zapper Toner

YIELD: ABOUT 1½ CUPS

1½ cups witch hazel tincture or commercial witch hazel

1 teaspoon dried peppermint leaves

1 teaspoon dried rosemary

1 teaspoon dried sage

3 to 5 drops echinacea extract

1 drop camphor essential oil

1 drop tea tree essential oil

Infuse the witch hazel with the peppermint leaves, rosemary, sage, echinacea extract, and essential oils in a glass jar. Cover and macerate at room temperature for 2 days. Shake the contents daily. After 2 days, strain into a bottle and discard the herbs. Use twice a day on clean skin, applying with a saturated cotton pad, cotton ball, or washcloth. Pat the toner gently over the face and neck area and behind the ears. If the mixture seems too strong, dilute with water. Stored in a sealed dark-glass bottle and kept in a cool, dark place, Zit Zapper Toner will keep for 2 years. Keep out of direct sunlight.

Bed-Wetting Extract

½ cup fresh St. John's wort flowers and leaves

¼ cup fresh lemon balm leaves

2 tablespoons dried orange flowers

Vodka or brandy

Put the St. John's wort flowers and leaves, lemon balm leaves, and orange flowers in a 1-quart glass jar and cover with vodka. Seal with a lid and let sit at room temperature for 2 weeks. Strain and discard the herbs. Stored in a sealed dark-glass bottle and kept in a cool, dark place, Bed-Wetting Extract will keep for 6 months to 2 years. Keep out of direct sunlight.

DOSAGE:

- For children six to ten years of age: Give 10 to 15 drops before bedtime.
- For children eleven to fifteen years of age: Give 20 drops immediately before or after dinner.

Tea Blend Two

3 teaspoons dried St. John's wort flowers

2 teaspoons dried lemon balm leaves

1 teaspoon dried orange flowers

Combine all the ingredients in a jar or a container with a lid. To use, place 1 to 1 ½ teaspoons of the herb mixture in a cup. Pour in 1 cup of boiling water. Steep for 20 minutes. Strain and discard the herbs. Stored in an airtight container in a cool, dark place, Tea Blend Two (the dry mixture only) will keep for 1 year. Keep out of direct sunlight.

DOSAGE:

- For children three to five years of age: Give ½ cup at dinnertime.
- For children six year of age and older: Give 1 cup at dinnertime.

Plantain-Arnica Compress

YIELD: ABOUT 1 CUP

Do not use remedies containing arnica on broken skin, including scrapes.

1 cup lukewarm water
1 tablespoon plantain tincture
1 tablespoon dried arnica flowers

Combine all the ingredients in a small bowl. Stored in a sealed glass jar in the refrigerator, Plantain-Arnica Compress will keep for 24 to 48 hours.

Alternatively, replace the tincture with ½ cup plantain-arnica infusion: Pour 1 cup of boiling water over 1 teaspoon dried arnica flowers and 1 teaspoon plantain leaves and steep for 10 to 15 minutes. Strain and discard the arnica. Use immediately.

APPLICATION INSTRUCTIONS: For children two years of age and older: Use a washcloth to apply the mixture to the affected areas.

See also: **First-Aid Remedy,** page 161
Plantain Salve, page 174

BURNS

See: **First-Aid Remedy,** page 161
St. John's Wort Salve, page 164
Soothing Salve, page 175

Chicken Pox Gentle Skin Wash   YIELD: ABOUT 1 CUP

This wash is gentle and soothing. It has only four ingredients, so it can be made easily and quickly.

5 cups water

1 ounce dried calendula flowers

1 ounce dried plantain leaves

1 ounce dried rosemary leaves

Combine all the ingredients in a medium saucepan over medium-high heat and bring to a boil. Decrease the heat to medium-low and simmer gently for 5 minutes. Remove from the heat and steep for 20 minutes.

Strain and discard the herbs. Let the strained liquid cool to a comfortably warm temperature before applying to the skin. Stored in a sealed glass container in the refrigerator, Chicken Pox Gentle Skin Wash will keep for 48 hours.

APPLICATION INSTRUCTIONS: For children one year of age and older: Apply to lesions and let air-dry.

Poxies Soothing Skin Wash   YIELD: ABOUT 6 CUPS

This wash features lavender and peppermint, which help heal the skin and soothe the inflammation and itching.

¼ to ½ cup dried rose petals

¼ to ½ cup dried lavender flowers

¼ to ½ cup dried peppermint leaves

¼ to ½ cup rolled oats

4 cups boiling water

2 cups witch hazel tincture or commercial witch hazel

Combine the rose petals, lavender flowers, peppermint leaves, and rolled oats in a large bowl. Pour the boiling water over the mixture and steep at room temperature until cool. Strain and discard the herbs. Stir in the witch hazel. Stored in a large, sealed glass jar in the refrigerator, Poxies Soothing Skin Wash will keep for 24 to 48 hours.

APPLICATION INSTRUCTIONS: For children 18 months of age and older: Use as a skin wash, add it to compresses, or add it to bath water.

Cold and Flu Body Rub

YIELD: ABOUT 1 CUP

1 cup almond, apricot kernel, or grapeseed oil

2 ounces beeswax, grated

10 drops eucalyptus essential oil

5 drops tea tree essential oil

Heat the almond oil and beeswax in a double boiler over simmering water until the beeswax is melted. Remove from the heat and stir in the essential oils. Pour into salve pots, a double-walled jar, or a jam jar and cool completely. Stored in a sealed container in a cool, dry place, Cold and Flu Body Rub will keep for 2 years.

APPLICATION INSTRUCTIONS: For children two years of age and older: Use as a massage oil.

Family Vitamin- and-Mineral Powder

YIELD: ABOUT 7 CUPS

2 cups nutritional yeast flakes

2 cups raw sesame seeds

1 cup powdered kelp

1 cup powdered dulse

½ cup freshly ground black pepper

2 tablespoons powdered stinging nettle

2 tablespoons spirulina

2 tablespoons sea salt

Garlic powder

Combine all the ingredients in a large bowl, adding garlic powder to taste. Mix well. Stored in a large, sealed glass jar in the refrigerator, Family Vitamin-and-Mineral Powder will keep for 3 to 6 months.

APPLICATION INSTRUCTIONS: For children one year of age and older: Sprinkle on food, such as pasta and vegetables, to boost immunity.

Flu Preventer
Children's Toy Cleaner

YIELD: ABOUT 1 CUP

1 cup distilled white vinegar

25 drops lemon essential oil

10 drops tea tree essential oil

Combine all the ingredients in a spray bottle. Stored in a cool, dark place, Flu Preventer Children's Toy Cleaner will keep for 2 years. Keep out of direct sunlight.

APPLICATION INSTRUCTIONS: Use as a spray cleaner during flu season to clean toys, toilets, laundry, and doorknobs—anything that is handled or touched often or that may harbor flu germs.

Immunity Tonic Tea

YIELD: ABOUT 2 CUPS

1 teaspoon dried echinacea flowers and leaves

1 teaspoon dried astragalus root

½ teaspoon dried boneset leaves

½ teaspoon dried licorice root

2 cups boiling water

Put the echinacea flowers and leaves, astragalus root, boneset leaves, and licorice root in a small saucepan. Pour the boiling water over the mixture. Steep at room temperature until cool. Strain and discard the herbs. Stored in a sealed glass jar in the refrigerator, Immunity Tonic Tea will keep for 48 hours.

DOSAGE:

- For children two to three years of age: ¼ cup a day.
- For children four to five years of age: 1 cup a day.
- For children six to twelve years of age: up to 2 cups a day.

Immunity Tonic Tincture

5 tablespoons dried echinacea flowers and leaves

5 tablespoons dried astragalus root

3 tablespoons dried boneset leaves

3 tablespoons dried licorice root

Vodka or brandy

Put the echinacea flowers and leaves, astragalus root, boneset leaves, and licorice root in a 1-quart jar. Cover with vodka and seal tightly. Once a day, give the jar a gentle shake. Allow the mixture to macerate at room temperature for 3 to 6 weeks. Strain and discard the herbs. Stored in a sealed glass jar in a cool, dark place, Immunity Tonic Tincture will keep for 6 to 12 months.

DOSAGE:

- For children two to three years of age: 5 drops a day.
- For children four to five years of age: Up to 10 drops a day.
- For children six to twelve years of age: Up to 20 drops a day.

Rose Hips Fruit Leather

Depending on the variety, rose hips can contain between 1,500 and 2,500 milligrams of vitamin C per 100 grams.

2 cups dried seedless rose hips *(Rosa canina)*

1 tablespoon agave nectar

1 tablespoon lemon juice

½ cup water, as needed

Preheat the oven to 150 degrees F. Line a jelly roll pan with parchment paper.

Put the rose hips, agave nectar, and lemon juice in a food processor and process until smooth. With the machine running, slowly add the water to achieve a mushy consistency that is neither too wet nor too dry. Pour into the prepared pan and spread the mixture evenly to within 1 inch of the sides. Bake for 8 hours, or until the mixture is no longer sticky to the touch. (Alternatively, place in a food dehydrator. Follow the manufacturer's instructions for processing fruit leather.)

Roll up the fruit leather and the paper together while still warm. (The paper will keep the fruit leather from sticking to itself.) Cool completely. Unroll and cut into strips or rectangles.

To store, loosely roll the cut fruit leather in plastic wrap and put it in a glass jar, plastic container, or food tin with a tightly sealed cover. Rose Hips Fruit Leather will keep for 1 year in the refrigerator and up to 2 years in the freezer. With longer storage, the fruit leather might dry out and become brittle, but it will still be edible. Do not eat it if it is moldy.

DOSAGE: For children three years of age (or younger, if they can chew well) and older: Eat as desired.

Rose Hips Tea YIELD: 1 CUP

Rosa rugosa *and* R. canina *are the tastiest varieties of rose hips.*

> 1 teaspoon dried rose hips
> 1 cup boiling water

Put the rose hips in a small bowl or cup and cover with the boiling water. Steep at room temperature until cool. Strain and discard the rose hips. Stored in a sealed glass jar in the refrigerator, Rose Hips Tea will keep for 48 hours.

DOSAGE:

- For children two to six years of age: 1 cup a day, unsweetened or mixed with juice.
- For children seven years of age and older: 2 to 3 cups a day, unsweetened or mixed with juice.

Basil Tea

- 1 teaspoon fresh basil leaves
- 1 cup boiling water

Place the basil leaves in a small bowl or cup and cover with the boiling water. Steep at room temperature until cool. Strain and discard the basil leaves. Stored in a sealed glass jar in the refrigerator, Basil Tea will keep for 48 hours.

DOSAGE: For babies three months of age and older: 1 teaspoon, 1 or 2 times a day.

Catnip Tea

- 1 teaspoon dried catnip leaves
- 1 cup boiling water

Put the catnip leaves in a small bowl or cup and cover with the boiling water. Steep at room temperature until cool. Strain and discard the catnip leaves. Store in a sealed glass jar in the refrigerator, Catnip Tea will keep for 48 hours.

DOSAGE:

- For children six months to one year of age: ½ teaspoon, 2 or 3 times a day.
- For children one to two years of age: 1 teaspoon, 2 or 3 times a day.
- For children three to seven years of age: 1½ teaspoons, 2 or 3 times a day.

GRIPE WATER TEAS

Dill and fennel are common ingredients in gripe water tea, which is a traditional English formula for soothing babies. Some parents sweeten the tea, but I don't think this is necessary. If you do choose to sweeten it, use a minimal amount of sweetener and don't use honey or corn syrup. Babies cannot metabolize the botulism spores that honey sometimes contains. Corn syrup is not sterilized and may be a source of contamination. For breast-fed babies, try administering the tea from a little cup or with a syringe, teaspoon, or eyedropper.

Dill Gripe Water Tea

2 cups water

1 teaspoon whole dill seeds, caraway seeds, or cardamom seeds

Combine the water and dill seeds in a small saucepan over medium-high heat. Simmer for 20 minutes. Strain and discard the seeds. Cool to room temperature or until just slightly warm. Stored in a sealed glass jar in the refrigerator, Dill Gripe Water Tea will keep for 24 hours. Alternatively, freeze any remaining tea in ice cube trays and melt as needed.

DOSAGE:

- For babies up to three months of age: 20 drops just before bedtime plus another 20 drops if baby awakes with severe gas pains.
- For babies four to nine months of age: 1 teaspoon just before bedtime plus another 1 teaspoon if baby awakes with severe gas pains.
- For babies ten months of age and older: ¼ cup just before bedtime plus another ¼ cup if baby awakes with severe gas pains.

Fennel Gripe Water

1 teaspoon whole fennel seeds

1¼ cups boiling water

Crush the fennel seeds in a cup or small bowl. Pour the boiling water over the crushed seeds and steep for 20 minutes. Strain and discard the seeds. Cool to room temperature, or until just slightly warm. Stored in a sealed glass jar in the refrigerator, Fennel Gripe Water will keep for 24 hours.

DOSAGE:

- For babies three months to six months of age: Start with ½ teaspoon and increase by 1 teaspoon an hour, up to 3 tablespoons maximum dose, if necessary to provide relief. Then give the lowest dose required to maintain comfort, 1 to 2 times a day.
- For children six months to two years of age: Start with 3 tablespoons and increase by 1 teaspoon an hour, up to ¼ cup maximum dose, if necessary to provide relief. Then give the lowest dose required to maintain comfort.
- For children three years of age and older: ¼ to 1 cup, 1 to 2 times a day.

Fennel, Ginger, and Peppermint Gripe Water

YIELD: 4 CUPS

4 cups water

1 teaspoon whole fennel seeds

1 (¼-inch) slice fresh ginger, peeled

1 tablespoon chopped fresh peppermint leaves, or 1 teaspoon dried

Combine the water, fennel seeds, and ginger in a medium saucepan over medium-high heat. Cover and simmer for 20 minutes. Remove from the heat and add the peppermint. Cool to room temperature, or until just slightly warm. Stored in a sealed glass jar in the refrigerator, Fennel, Ginger, and Peppermint Gripe Water will keep for 24 hours.

DOSAGE:

- For children six months to one year of age: ½ teaspoon, 1 or 2 times a day.
- For children two to three years of age: 1 teaspoon, 1 or 2 times a day.
- For children four to seven years of age, 1½ teaspoons, 1 or 2 times a day.

CONJUNCTIVITIS

About Eyewashes

To avoid contagion or introducing new germs, it's absolutely imperative that all equipment used in making and administering eyewashes be sterilized. Even the water for the decoctions should be boiled for at least ten minutes before being used in the recipes. In addition, be sure to sterilize the eyecup or eyedropper for ten minutes in boiling water before each use, and do not use the same eyecup on both eyes without sterilizing it again.

Strain the eyewashes thoroughly—through a piece of cheesecloth, gauze or a clean coffee filter—to remove the herbs.

Apply eyewash by pouring it over the eye or by moistening a cotton ball with the eyewash and dabbing it onto the child's eye. For older children, use an eyecup or compress.

The first application of any eyewash should be done first thing in the morning; the last should be right before bed. For very irritated eyes, use a compress two to three times per day instead of, or in addition to, the second eyewash of the day.

Using an Eyecup

To use an eyecup, fill it with the eyewash. Holding it level, lower your head so your eye is inside the eyecup and immersed in the eyewash. Open your eye and roll it around and blink a few times so that the eyewash is distributed over the entire eye area. Do this for one minute.

Using a Compress

To make a compress, use a cotton pad or clean cotton cloth. Submerge the cloth in the eyewash and squeeze to remove excess liquid. Place the compress on the eye for at least 10 minutes at a time.

CAUTION: Never take undiluted tincture straight out of the bottle and put it directly into the eye.

Eyebright Eyewash   YIELD: 1 CUP

> 1 teaspoon dried eyebright flowers or leaves
> 1 cup boiling water

Put the eyebright in a cup or small bowl. Boil the water for at least 10 minutes before pouring it over the eyebright. Steep until completely cool. Strain and discard the eyebright. (See Using an Eyecup, page 145.) Stored in a sealed glass jar in the refrigerator, Eyebright Eyewash will keep for 48 hours.

VARIATION: Pour the boiling water into a cup or small bowl. Cool completely. Substitute 1 teaspoon of eyebright tincture and add it to the cooled water.

CAUTION: Never take undiluted tincture straight out of the bottle and put it directly into the eye.

APPLICATION INSTRUCTIONS: For children five years of age and older: Apply 2 to 3 times a day using an eyecup or a cotton ball.

Goldenseal Eyewash

2 heaping teaspoons boric acid

1 teaspoon dried goldenseal flowers

½ teaspoon myrrh powder

2 cups boiling water

½ cup water

Put the boric acid, goldenseal flowers, and myrrh powder in a small bowl. Boil the 2 cups of water for at least 10 minutes before pouring it over them. Steep until completely cool. Strain and discard the solids. To make the eyewash, add 1 teaspoon of the strained liquid to ½ cup water. Stored in a sealed glass jar in the refrigerator, Goldenseal Eyewash will keep for 48 hours.

APPLICATION INSTRUCTIONS: For children five years of age and older: Apply 1 to 2 times a day, or up to 3 times a day, if needed, using an eyecup or a cotton ball.(See Using an Eyecup, page 145.)

Purple Loosestrife Eyewash

1 teaspoon dried purple loosestrife flowers

1 cup boiling water

Put the purple loosestrife flowers in a small bowl. Boil the water for at least 10 minutes before pouring it over the loosestrife. Steep until completely cool. Strain and discard the flowers. Stored in a sealed glass jar in the refrigerator, Purple Loosestrife Eyewash will keep for 48 hours.

VARIATIONS: Substitute 1 teaspoon dried lady's mantle flowers, dried red raspberry leaves, or dried meadowsweet flowers for the loosestrife flowers.

APPLICATION INSTRUCTIONS: For children three years of age and older: Apply 3 times a day, using an eyecup or a cotton ball. (See Using an Eyecup, page 145.)

Three-Flower Eyewash

1 teaspoon dried calendula flowers

1 teaspoon dried chamomile flowers

1 teaspoon dried eyebright flowers

3 cups boiling water

Put the calendula, chamomile, and eyebright flowers in a bowl. Boil the water for at least 10 minutes before pouring it over the flowers. Steep until completely cool. Strain, reserving both the liquid and the flowers separately. Stored in a sealed glass jar in the refrigerator, Three-Flower Eyewash will keep for 48 hours.

APPLICATION INSTRUCTIONS:

- For children three years of age and older: Put the reserved flowers in a clean washcloth and use as a compress 2 to 3 times a day, or as often as needed.

- For children five years of age and older: Apply the strained liquid 2 to 3 times a day, using an eyecup or a cotton ball. (See Using an Eyecup, page 145.)

Cough and Throat Drops

YIELD: 30 TO 60 COUGH DROPS

1 to 2 teaspoons dried angelica root

1 to 2 teaspoons dried coltsfoot leaves

1 to 2 teaspoons dried echinacea flowers

1 to 2 teaspoons dried elder flowers

1 to 2 teaspoons dried elecampane root

1 to 2 teaspoons dried horehound or comfrey leaves

1 to 2 teaspoons dried marshmallow root

1 to 2 teaspoons dried mullein leaves

1 to 2 teaspoons dried sage leaves

1 to 2 teaspoons dried thyme leaves

4 cups water

2 cups turbinado sugar

¾ cup light corn syrup

⅛ teaspoon peppermint, eucalyptus, or anise essential oil

Oil a baking sheet and set aside.

Combine the angelica root, coltsfoot leaves, echinacea flowers, elder flowers, elecampane root, horehound leaves, marshmallow root, mullein leaves, sage leaves, and thyme leaves in a large saucepan. To make a strong decoction, add the water and simmer over medium-high heat until the liquid has reduced to 1 cup.

Stir in the sugar and corn syrup. Simmer over medium heat, stirring constantly, until the sugar dissolves. Decrease the heat to low and simmer without stirring for 20 to 30 minutes, until the mixture reaches hard-ball candy stage (300 degrees F on a candy thermometer). Remove the pan from the heat and stir in the essential oil. Immediately pour the mixture onto the prepared baking sheet. With the back of a spoon, smooth it to about ½-inch thick. Let cool.

The syrup will begin to harden immediately. When it is cool enough to handle, pull up the edges and cut the mixture into strips with scissors. Snip the strips into lozenge-size pieces. Alternatively, break off pieces by hand as the mixture cools. Stored in an airtight container, Cough and Throat Drops will keep for 2 years.

DOSAGE: For children five years of age and older: 1 cough drop dissolved in the mouth, 4 to 5 times a day.

Variation: To make a Cough and Throat Tea, make a decoction using 1 tablespoon dried thyme leaves, 1 tablespoon dried licorice root, 1 tablespoon dried sage leaves, 1 tablespoon whole anise seeds (*Pimpinella anisum,* not star anise), and 2 cups of water. If the cough is causing your child to hack and stay up at night, add 2 tablespoons wild cherry bark. Stored in a sealed glass jar in the refrigerator, Cough and Throat Tea will keep for 48 hours. Give the tea before bedtime.

DOSAGE:

- For children two to three years of age: ½ cup.
- For children four to six years of age: 1 cup.
- For children age six and older: Up to 2 cups.

Elderberry Cough Syrup
YIELD: 2 TO 3 CUPS

6 cups fresh elderberries

⅓ cup honey or vegetable glycerin

1 teaspoon dried marshmallow root

1 teaspoon boneset leaves, echinacea flowers or root, or licorice root

¼ teaspoon ground cinnamon

2 cups vodka or brandy

1 tablespoon lime or lemon juice

Mash the elderberries in a large strainer over a bowl, capturing the juice in the bowl. Transfer the juice to a medium saucepan and add the honey, marshmallow, boneset, and cinnamon. Cover and simmer over medium heat for 35 minutes. Remove from the heat and stir in the vodka and lime juice. Strain and discard the herbs. Cool thoroughly. Stored in a sealed glass bottle in the refrigerator, Elderberry Cough Syrup will keep for 1 year.

DOSAGE:

- For babies birth to fourteen months of age: Seek medical advice.
- For babies six to fourteen months of age: 1 to 2 teaspoons per day.
- For children fifteen months to three years of age: 2 to 4 teaspoons per day.
- For children four years of age and older: 2 to 4 tablespoons per day.

Lemon Cough Syrup

This syrup is potent and is most appropriate for children two years of age or older. It helps break up congestion in the lungs and soothes a sore throat.

> 1 medium onion, minced
>
> 1¼ cups honey or agave nectar
>
> 3 to 5 drops lemon, peppermint, or tea tree essential oil

Put the onion in a shallow bowl and pour the honey over it. Cover and set aside at room temperature for 8 to 12 hours. Strain and discard the onion. Add the essential oil to the strained liquid and mix well. Stored in a sealed glass bottle in the refrigerator, Lemon Cough Syrup will keep for 3 to 6 months.

DOSAGE:

- For children two to six years of age: 2 teaspoons in herbal tea or hot water, 2 to 3 times a day.
- For children seven years of age and older: 1 tablespoon in herbal tea or hot water, 2 to 3 times a day.

Vermont Cough Syrup

2 tablespoons dried peppermint leaves
2 tablespoons dried slippery elm bark
2 tablespoons dried valerian root
2 tablespoons dried chamomile flowers
1 tablespoon echinacea root
1 tablespoon goldenseal root
1 tablespoon dried hops flowers
1 tablespoon dried mullein leaves
1 tablespoon dried coltsfoot leaves
1 tablespoon dried eucalyptus leaves
1 tablespoon dried licorice root
1 tablespoon chopped fresh ginger root
20 drops eucalyptus essential oil
4 cups water, plus more as needed
½ cup honey
¼ cup vodka or brandy
10 to 15 drops peppermint essential oil

Combine the peppermint leaves, slippery elm bark, valerian root, chamomile flowers, echinacea root, goldenseal root, hops flowers, mullein leaves, coltsfoot leaves, eucalyptus leaves, licorice root, ginger root, and eucalyptus essential oil in a large nonmetallic saucepan. Pour in the water, or enough to cover by about 2 inches, and bring to a boil. Decrease the heat and simmer for 30 minutes, adding water as necessary to keep the mixture from scorching. Remove from the heat and steep for 1 hour.

Strain the mixture through a piece of cheesecloth and discard the solids. Rinse out the saucepan and return the strained liquid to the pan. Stir in the honey and vodka. Bring to a boil, stirring constantly. Decrease the heat to medium-low and simmer, stirring constantly, until syrupy. Pour into 2 (2-quart) jars or bottles, filling them only about three-quarters full. Divide the peppermint oil equally between the jars, cover, and shake well. Stored in the sealed glass jars in the refrigerator, Vermont Cough Syrup will keep for 3 to 6 months.

DOSAGE:

- For children two to six years of age: 1 to 3 teaspoons, 2 or 3 times a day.
- For children seven years of age and older: 1 to 2 tablespoons, 2 or 3 times a day.

Wild Cherry Cough Syrup

1 cup water

2 tablespoons wild cherry bark (optional)

1 tablespoon dried thyme

1 tablespoon licorice root

1 tablespoon dried sage leaves

1 tablespoon whole anise seeds

1 cup plus 2 to 3 tablespoons honey

Combine the water, optional wild cherry bark, thyme, licorice root, sage, and anise seeds in a medium saucepan. Bring to a boil over medium-high heat. Decrease the heat to medium-low and simmer for 20 minutes.

Remove from the heat and strain the mixture through a piece of cheesecloth. Discard the solids. Rinse out the saucepan and return the strained liquid to the pan. Stir in the honey. Simmer for 30 minutes, stirring almost constantly. Remove from the heat. Cool completely. Stored in a sealed glass bottle in the refrigerator, Wild Cherry Cough Syrup will keep for 3 months.

NOTE: Add the wild cherry bark for a hacking, nighttime cough. The syrup will keep for 1 or 2 months longer if you add 2 to 3 more tablespoons of honey and 2 to 3 tablespoons of vodka or brandy.

DOSAGE:

- For children two to six years of age: 1 to 3 teaspoons a day.
- For children seven years of age and older: 1 tablespoon, as needed, up to 4 times a day.

Cradle Cap Blend

YIELD: ABOUT ½ CUP

Dried or fresh calendula flowers
Dried or fresh chamomile flowers
½ cup olive oil

Pack a 1-pint jar with the calendula and chamomile flowers and pour the oil over them. Cover and set aside for 2 weeks at room temperature. Strain and discard the flowers. Pour the strained oil into a glass jar. Stored in a sealed glass jar in a cool, dry place, Cradle Cap Blend will keep for 6 months.

APPLICATION INSTRUCTIONS: For babies two months of age and older: Apply to the scalp 2 to 3 times a day, or as needed.

Bum-Bum Powder

YIELD: ABOUT 2 CUPS

1 cup fine white or pink clay
½ cup cornstarch
2 tablespoons black walnut hull powder
2 tablespoons myrrh powder
1 tablespoon goldenseal powder
1 or 2 drops tea tree essential oil

Combine all the ingredients in a large bowl. Stored in a sealed container at room temperature, Bum-Bum Powder will keep for 1 year.

APPLICATION INSTRUCTIONS: For babies two months of age and older: For constant barrier protection or to protect sensitive skin, use after every diaper change or when a rash is present.

Jacob's Salve

2 teaspoons St. John's wort flowers

2 teaspoons calendula petals

2 teaspoons plantain leaves

2 teaspoons comfrey leaves

2 teaspoons echinacea leaves

½ cup olive oil

2 tablespoons beeswax, grated

15 drops vitamin E oil

Several drops lavender essential oil

Following the directions for making infused oil on pages 117–118, prepare an infused oil using the flowers, petals, leaves, and olive oil.

To make a salve, melt the beeswax in a small saucepan over medium-low heat. Stir in the infused oil, vitamin E oil, and lavender essential oil. Pour into salve pots, and set aside until firm. Stored in sealed salve pots at room temperature, Jacob's Salve will keep for 2 years.

NOTE: Vitamin E oil is generally available in two strengths—32,000 IU and 45,000 IU. Either strength can be used in this recipe.

APPLICATION INSTRUCTIONS: For babies two months of age and older: Apply at every diaper change.

Goldenseal Salve

4 tablespoons dried comfrey leaves

4 tablespoons dried calendula flowers

2 tablespoons goldenseal root powder

1 teaspoon myrrh powder

2 cups olive oil

¼ to ½ cup grated beeswax

15 drops vitamin E oil

Following the directions for making infused oil on pages 117–118, prepare an infused oil using the leaves, flowers, powders, and olive oil.

To make a salve, melt the beeswax in a small saucepan over medium-low heat. Stir in the infused oil and the vitamin E oil. Pour into salve pots, and set aside until firm. Stored in sealed salve pots at room temperature, Goldenseal Salve will keep for 2 years.

NOTE: Vitamin E oil is generally available in two strengths—32,000 IU and 45,000 IU. Either strength can be used in this recipe.

APPLICATION INSTRUCTIONS: For babies one month to three years of age: For bad rashes, use for every diaper change.

Taro's Bummi Cream

YIELD: ABOUT 1½ CUPS

This is a strong and effective salve for diaper rash.

½ cup almond oil

½ cup olive oil

½ cup cocoa butter

2 tablespoons coconut oil

1 cup fresh mashed calendula flowers

1 cup mashed dried or fresh chamomile flowers

¼ cup grated beeswax (optional)

Combine the almond oil, olive oil, cocoa butter, and coconut oil in a double boiler over simmering water until the cocoa butter has melted. Remove the pan from the double boiler and set aside to cool for 5 minutes. Mash the calendula and chamomile flowers in a bowl. Gently stir them into the oil mixture. Cover and set aside for 8 to 12 hours.

Heat the mixture in a double boiler over simmering water, adding the beeswax if the salve is too soft. Strain the mixture through a fine sieve, clean tea towel, or piece of cheesecloth and discard the herbs. (It's all right to leave fine pieces of the flowers in the salve.) Stir and pour into salve pots. Let stand at room temperature until set. Stored in sealed salve pots at room temperature, Taro's Bummi Cream will keep for 2 years.

APPLICATION INSTRUCTIONS: For babies two months of age and older: Apply to affected area as needed. Discontinue use if irritation occurs.

See also: **Plantain Salve, page 174**

Homemade Ginger Tea

YIELD: 1 CUP

1 (¼-inch) slice fresh ginger

1 cup boiling water

Put the ginger in a cup and pour the boiling water over it. Steep until cool. Discard the ginger.

DOSAGE:

- For children eight months to two years of age: 1 to 2 teaspoons a day.
- For children three to seven years of age: 2 to 4 tablespoons a day.
- For children eight years of age and older: 1 to 2 cups a day.

Slippery Elm Gruel

YIELD: ABOUT 2 CUPS

1½ teaspoon slippery elm bark powder

¼ cup cold water or juice

2 cups water, apple juice, or grape juice

Combine the slippery elm bark powdeer and cold water in a small cup or bowl and stir to make a paste. Set aside.

Put the water in a small saucepan and bring to a boil over medium-high heat. Add the paste, decrease the heat to medium-low, and simmer, whisking constantly, for 2 minutes. Serve warm.

DOSAGE:

- For children eight months to one year of age: 1 to 2 teaspoons.
- For children one to two years of age: 1 to 2 tablespoons.
- For children three to four years of age: 3 to 5 tablespoons.
- For children five to six years of age: 5 to 6 tablespoons.
- For children seven to eight years of age: 7 to 8 tablespoons.
- For children nine to twelve years of age: 1 cup.
- For children thirteen years of age and older: 1 to 2 cups.

VARIATIONS: To vary the flavor, add a little grated lemon rind or spices (such as ground cinnamon, cloves, or nutmeg) to taste. For children older than two years of age, a little honey and a small amount of dried fruit (such as raisins or chopped dates or apricots) may be added if they can be chewed safely.

Achy Ear Oil

YIELD: ABOUT ½ CUP

½ cup fresh mullein flowers

¼ cup fresh St. John's wort flowers

½ cup olive oil

2 cloves garlic, peeled and sliced

Following the directions for making infused oil on pages 117–118, pre-pare an infused oil using the flowers, oil, and garlic. Stored in glass dropper bottles in a cool, dry place, Achy Ear Oil will keep for 3 to 6 months.

DOSAGE: For children three months of age and older: 2 drops in each ear, 2 or 3 times a day.

Black Walnut Salve

YIELD: ABOUT 4 (4-ounce) CONTAINERS

¼ cup infused black walnut oil

¼ cup infused chaparral oil

¼ cup infused myrrh oil

¼ cup infused burdock oil

¼ cup infused echinacea oil

1 cup grated beeswax

30 drops vitamin E oil

To make a salve, heat the infused oils in a small saucepan over medium-low heat until warm. Add the beeswax. After the beeswax melts, remove from the heat. Set aside to cool for 5 minutes. Stir in the vita-min E oil.

Pour into salve pots, and set aside until firm. Stored in sealed salve pots at room temperature, Black Walnut Salve will keep for 2 years.

NOTE: Vitamin E oil is generally available in two strengths—32,000 IU and 45,000 IU. Either strength can be used in this recipe.

APPLICATION INSTRUCTIONS: For children six months of age and older: Apply Black Wal-nut Salve 3 to 4 times a day, as needed. Discontinue if irritation develops.

Eczema Tea

1 teaspoon dried lemon balm leaves

1 teaspoon dried red clover flowers

1 teaspoon dried stinging nettle leaves

1 cup boiling water

Put the lemon balm leaves, red clover flowers, and stinging nettle leaves in a cup. Pour the boiling water over the herbs and steep until lukewarm. Strain and discard the herbs. Stored in a sealed glass jar in the refrigerator, Eczema Tea will keep for 48 hours.

DOSAGE AND APPLICATION INSTRUCTIONS:

- For children three years of age or older: 1 cup of the tea, 2 to 3 times a day.
- For children six months of age and older: Apply topically in a compress.

See also: **Calendula Salve,** page 174

Soothing Salve, page 175

Goldenseal Salve, page 154

Plantain Salve, page 174

FUNGAL INFECTIONS

See: **Black Walnut Salve,** page 157

St. John's Wort Salve, page 164

HAND, FOOT, AND MOUTH DISEASE

Anti-Gel

1 cup aloe vera gel

2 tablespoons vodka

30 drops tea tree essential oil

Combine all the ingredients in a glass container with a lid and shake to mix well. Stored in a sealed container in the refrigerator, Anti-Gel will keep for 6 months.

APPLICATION INSTRUCTIONS:

- For children younger than one year of age: Dilute 1 tablespoon Anti-Gel with 1½ teaspoons water before applying. Apply 2 to 3 times a day.
- For children one to two years of age: Apply undiluted 2 to 3 times a day.
- For children three years of age and older: Apply undiluted 3 to 4 times a day.

HEADACHES

Headache Tea
YIELD: 1 CUP

1 teaspoon dried peppermint leaves
1 teaspoon dried or fresh rosemary leaves
1 teaspoon dried or fresh chamomile flowers
1 teaspoon dried or fresh lavender flowers
1 cup boiling water

Put the peppermint leaves, rosemary leaves, chamomile flowers, and lavender flowers in a cup. Pour the boiling water over the herbs and steep until lukewarm. Strain and discard the herbs. Stored in a sealed glass jar in the refrigerator, Headache Tea will keep for 48 hours.

DOSAGE: For children four years of age and older: 1 cup, 2 to 3 times a day, as needed.

Headache Tincture
YIELD: VARIES WITH QUANTITY MADE

1 part dried or fresh lavender flowers
1 part dried or fresh skullcap flowers or leaves
1 part rolled oats

Prepare a tincture in a 1-quart jar using equal amounts of lavender flowers, skullcap flowers or leaves, and rolled oats. Stored in a sealed glass bottle in a cool, dark place, Headache Tincture will keep for 1 year.

DOSAGE: For children five years of age and older: Follow the tincture dosage guidelines on page 64.

Mild Head Lice Oil

YIELD: ½ CUP OIL

1/2 cup olive oil

FOR CHILDREN THREE YEARS OF AGE AND OLDER: 30 to 40 drops eucalyptus, geranium, lavender, or tea tree essential oil

FOR CHILDREN SEVEN YEARS OF AGE AND OLDER: 30 to 40 drops ginger, rosemary, or thyme essential oil

Combine the olive oil with one of the essential oils in a jar with a lid or other covered container, using the appropriate amount for your child's age. Stored in a sealed container in a cool, dark place, Mild Head Lice Oil will keep for 6 months.

APPLICATION INSTRUCTIONS: For children three years of age and older: Rub Mild Head Lice Oil into the scalp. Use enough to saturate the head and all of the hair, but do not get it into the eyes. Cover the child's hair with a bathing cap or plastic wrap and leave on for 12 hours or overnight. Wash the hair with Tea Tree Shampoo (page 161), using 2 to 3 drops of tea tree essential oil. Comb the hair with a nit comb to remove the head lice.

TIP: Perform the nit-combing ritual in direct sunlight so you can see what you're doing. If the nit comb isn't working, "strip" out the nits by hand, carefully moving from one section of hair to another. You might have to repeat this daily until you can no longer find any newly hatched nits.

Lice Leavers Oil

YIELD: 1 APPLICATION

1/2 cup jojoba oil

2 tablespoons coconut oil

15 drops chamomile essential oil

15 drops tea tree essential oil

15 drops oregano essential oil

Combine the jojoba oil, coconut oil, and essential oils in a jar with a lid or other covered container. Stored in a covered container in a cool, dark place, Lice Leavers Oil will keep for 2 to 3 weeks.

For children five years of age and older: Rub Lice Leavers Oil into the scalp. Use enough to saturate the head and all the hair, but do not get it into the eyes. Cover your child's hair with a bathing cap or plastic wrap and leave on for 12 hours or overnight. Wash the hair with Tea Tree Shampoo (page 161), using 3 to 5 drops of tea tree essential oil. Comb the hair with a nit comb to remove the head lice. (See the tip on page 160.)

Tea Tree Shampoo
YIELD: ½ CUP SHAMPOO

2 to 5 drops tea tree or oregano essential oil

4 ounces all-natural shampoo .

Make Tea Tree Shampoo just before using. Add the tea tree essential oil to the shampoo and stir to mix well.

INSECT BITES AND STINGS

First-Aid Remedy
YIELD: ABOUT 2 TABLESPOONS

3 drops lavender essential oil

3 drops tea tree essential oil

3 drops German chamomile essential oil

3 drops helichrysum essential oil

2 tablespoons calendula infused oil

Combine all the ingredients in a small bowl. Stored in a sealed dark-glass jar with an orifice reducer, First-Aid Remedy will keep for 2 years.

APPLICATION INSTRUCTIONS: For children five years of age and older: Dab onto affected areas as needed.

NOTE: German chamomile essential oil is gentler than regular chamomile essential oil, which can cause reactions.

Clay Poultice

As the clay mixture dries on the skin, it pulls toxins and pus from stings and bites to keep the pain from spreading.

 1 tablespoon bentonite clay

 1 teaspoon echinacea root tincture

 1 teaspoon chamomile tincture

 1 teaspoon plantain tincture

 12 drops lavender essential oil

Put the clay in the container the poultice will be stored in. Gradually add the tinctures, stirring between each addition so the clay absorbs the liquid. Sprinkle with the lavender oil, stirring to distribute it evenly in the clay mixture. Covered tightly and stored at room temperature, Clay Poultice will keep for 3 to 4 months. If the clay dries out, sprinkle it with a little distilled water to reconstitute it.

APPLICATION INSTRUCTIONS: For children ten years of age and older: Dab onto the affected areas, allow to dry, and wipe off with warm water.

Cootie Oil

 ¼ cup almond, olive, or apricot kernel oil

 10 drops linalol essential oil

 5 drops lavender essential oil

 5 drops rosemary essential oil

 3 drops lemon essential oil

 1 drop clove bud essential oil

 1 drop cinnamon bark essential oil

Combine all the ingredients in a mister bottle or in a bottle with an orifice reducer. Stored in sealed dark-glass bottle in a cool, dark place, Cootie Oil will keep for 8 to 12 months.

APPLICATION INSTRUCTIONS: For children five years of age and older: Dab onto insect bites as needed, 3 to 5 times a day. If using a mister bottle, spray in the air and walk through the mist or apply lightly to body. If using a bottle with an orifice reducer, apply to wrists, ankles, neck, and backs of the knees.

NOTE: Cootie Oil will stain clothing.

Insect-Aside Bug Repellent

¼ cup olive, almond, or apricot kernel oil

8 drops cedar essential oil

5 drops eucalyptus essential oil

4 drops lavender essential oil

2 drops orange essential oil

2 drops lemon essential oil

1 drop peppermint essential oil

1 drop clove essential oil

1 drop cinnamon essential oil

Combine all the ingredients in a 5- or 6-ounce glass bottle with a lid and shake to mix well. Stored in a sealed dark-glass bottle in a cool, dry place, Insect-Aside Bug Repellent will keep for 2 years. Shake well before each use.

APPLICATION INSTRUCTIONS: For children five years of age and older: Shake well before using. Apply liberally to exposed skin 3 to 4 times a day. Keep away from the eyes.

Insect Bite Gel

1 teaspoon aloe vera gel

5 drops lavender or tea tree essential oil

Combine the aloe vera gel and essential oil in a roll-on stick. Sealed tightly and stored in the refrigerator, Insect Bite Gel will keep for 8 months.

APPLICATION INSTRUCTIONS: For children 10 months of age and older: Apply to insect bites every few hours to soothe and relieve soreness.

St. John's Wort Salve

1 cup St. John's wort flowers

1 cup calendula flowers

1 cup comfrey leaves

1 cup grated beeswax

1 (400 IU) vitamin E capsule

Following the directions for making infused oil on pages 117–118, prepare an infused oil using the St. John's wort, calendula, and comfrey.

To make a salve, melt the beeswax in a small saucepan over medium-low heat. Stir in the infused oil and the oil from the vitamin E capsule. Pour into salve pots, and set aside until firm. Stored in sealed salve pots at room temperature, St. John's Wort Salve will keep for 2 years.

APPLICATION INSTRUCTIONS: For children six months of age and older: Rub a small amount on the affected area 2 to 5 times a day.

MENSTRUAL PROBLEMS

Cramping-Up Tea

YIELD: ABOUT 3 CUPS

This high-calcium tea helps ease painful menstrual periods.

1 tablespoon dried cramp bark

1 tablespoon dried red raspberry leaves

1 tablespoon dried stinging nettle leaves

1 teaspoon dried comfrey leaves

1 teaspoon dried oat straw

3 cups boiling water

Combine the cramp bark, red raspberry leaves, stinging nettle leaves, comfrey leaves, and oat straw in a medium bowl. Add the boiling water and steep for 15 minutes. Strain and discard the herbs. Stored in a sealed glass jar in the refrigerator, Cramping-Up Tea will keep for 48 hours.

DOSAGE: For teen girls: 1 cup, 2 or 3 times a day.

Cypress Oil Massage Blend YIELD: ABOUT 4 OUNCES

4 ounces almond oil, apricot kernel oil, or olive oil

10 drops cypress essential oil

10 drops geranium essential oil

10 drops lemon essential oil

10 drops roman chamomile essential oil

Combine the almond oil and essential oils in a cup or small container. Stored in a sealed dark-glass bottle in a cool, dark place, Cypress Oil Massage Blend will keep for about 15 months.

APPLICATION INSTRUCTIONS: Massage into the abdomen 3 times a day or as needed. Do not use if the skin is already irritated or becomes irritated with use.

IronWomyn YIELD: VARIES WITH QUANTITY MADE

2 parts stinging nettle tincture

2 parts dandelion root tincture

2 parts dandelion leaf tincture

1 part yellow dock root tincture

1 part red raspberry leaf tincture

Combine all the tinctures in a bowl. Stored in a glass dropper bottle in a cool, dry place, IronWomyn will keep for 1 to 2 years.

DOSAGE:

- For teen girls, three days *before* the period is expected: 30 drops straight or in water, 3 to 4 times a day.
- For teen girls, two to three days *after* menstruation: 30 drops straight or in water, 2 to 3 times a day or as needed to replenish iron in the blood due to heavy menstrual periods.

EASY RECIPES FOR HOMEMADE REMEDIES **165**

Menstrual Cramp Oil

YIELD: ABOUT 1 OUNCE

2 tablespoons almond oil, apricot kernel oil, or olive oil

4 drops lavender essential oil

3 drops geranium essential oil

2 drops chamomile essential oil

2 drops marjoram essential oil

1 drop ginger essential oil

1 drop patchouli essential oil

Combine the almond oil and essential oils in a cup or small container. Stored in a sealed dark-glass bottle in a cool, dark place, Menstrual Cramp Oil will keep for 1 year.

APPLICATION INSTRUCTIONS: Use to massage the abdomen and hips.

Periwinkle Blend

YIELD: 3 TABLESPOONS

1 cup water

1 tablespoon dried american cranesbill root

1 tablespoon beth root

1 tablespoon periwinkle leaves

Combine all the ingredients in a small saucepan and simmer over medium heat for 20 minutes. Remove from the heat and steep for 20 to 30 minutes. Strain and discard the solids. Stored in a sealed glass jar in the refrigerator, Periwinkle Blend will keep for 48 hours.

DOSAGE: For teen girls: 1 cup, 3 times a day before and during the menstrual period, with health-care guidance. If desired, sweeten with honey or stevia to taste.

Profuse Menstruation Regulation Blend

YIELD: ABOUT 3 CUPS

3 cups of water

2 teaspoons dried yellow dock root

2 teaspoons dried red raspberry leaves

2 teaspoons dried stinging nettle leaves

Bring the water to a boil in a medium saucepan. Add the yellow dock root and simmer for 20 minutes. Remove from the heat and stir in the red raspberry leaves and stinging nettle leaves. Steep for 20 minutes. Strain and discard the solids. Stored in a sealed glass jar in the refrigerator, Profuse Menstruation Regulation Blend will keep for 48 hours.

DOSAGE: For teen girls: 1 cup, 2 or 3 times a day.

Severe Cramp Extract   YIELD: VARIES WITH QUANTITY MADE

- 1 part cramp bark extract
- 1 part motherwort extract
- 1 part wild yam extract

Combine all the extracts in a small bowl. Stored in a glass dropper bottle in a cool, dry place, Severe Cramp Extract will keep for 1 to 2 years.

DOSAGE: For teen girls: In an acute situation, administer up to 30 drops every 10 minutes until the cramping subsides.

Spasm Massage Oil   YIELD: ABOUT 1 OUNCE

- 10 drops peppermint essential oil
- 5 drops clary sage essential oil
- 5 drops cypress essential oil
- 5 drops lavender essential oil

Combine all the ingredients in a cup or small bowl. Stored in a sealed glass bottle in a cool, dry place, Spasm Massage Oil will keep for 1 to 2 years.

APPLICATION INSTRUCTIONS: Use to massage pelvis, hips, and buttocks, or add a few drops to a warm bath or sitz bath.

Motion Sickness Blend   YIELD: ENOUGH FOR DOZENS OF DOSAGES

This remedy also works for adults who get carsick—adults can take the same dosage as older children.

- ½ cup dried chamomile flowers
- ¼ cup dried peppermint leaves
- ¼ cup dried lemon balm leaves
- 2 tablespoons dried hops flowers

Combine all the ingredients in a medium bowl and mix well. Stored in a sealed jar at room temperature, Motion Sickness Blend will keep for 6 months. To use, add 2 tablespoons of the mixture to 1 cup boiling water and steep for 15 minutes. Strain and discard the herbs. Give the first dose about 30 minutes to 1 hour before a trip.

DOSAGE:

- For babies six months to two years of age: Seek medical advice.
- For children three to five years of age: ½ cup, 1 to 2 times a day.
- For children six years of age and older: Up to 2 cups a day.

Muscle-Easing Liniment   YIELD: 1 TO 4 APPLICATIONS

- ½ cup vodka
- 1 teaspoon peppermint, eucalyptus, or rosemary essential oil

Combine the vodka and essential oil in a clean, dry jar. Cover tightly and shake well to mix. Stored at room temperature, Muscle-Easting Liniment will keep for 6 months.

APPLICATION INSTRUCTIONS: For children six years of age and older: Apply to strains, pains, and sports injuries 3 to 5 times a day.

Garlic Honey

¼ cup honey

1 clove garlic, crushed with the flat side of a knife

Combine the honey and garlic in a cup or small bowl. Cover and refrigerate or let stand at room temperature for 3 to 5 days. Remove and discard the garlic.

Alternatively, warm the honey and garlic together in a small saucepan. Remove from the heat and set aside until completely cool. Remove and discard the garlic. Stored in a sealed glass jar, Garlic Honey will keep for 3 months at room temperature or 6 months in the refrigerator.

DOSAGE: For children two years of age and older: 1 teaspoon straight or in a cup of herbal tea, 2 to 3 times a day.

NOTE: Honey should not be given to children younger than two years of age.

Super Sinus-Clearing Tea

3 to 6 tablespoons dried usnea

3 to 6 tablespoons echinacea root

3 to 6 tablespoons dried hibiscus flowers

3 cups boiling water

Combine the usnea, echinacea root, and hibiscus flowers in a bowl. Add the boiling water and steep for 15 to 20 minutes. Strain and discard the solids. Serve warm. Stored in a sealed glass jar in the refrigerator, Super Sinus-Clearing Tea will keep for 48 hours.

DOSAGE:

- For children two to four years of age: ¼ cup, 2 to 3 times a day.
- For children five to eight years of age: ½ cup, 2 to 3 times a day.
- For children nine to twelve years of age: 1 cup, 2 to 3 times a day.
- For children thirteen years of age and older: 1 cup, 3 times a day.

Echinacea Sinus Tea

YIELD: 3 CUPS

3 to 6 tablespoons dried lemon balm leaves

3 to 6 tablespoons dried echinacea root

3 to 6 tablespoons dried rose hips

3 cups boiling water

Combine the lemon balm, echinacea, and rose hips in a bowl. Add the boiling water and steep for 30 minutes. Strain and discard the solids. Serve warm. Stored in a sealed glass jar in the refrigerator, Echinacea Sinus Tea will keep for 48 hours.

DOSAGE: For children six years of age and older: 2 to 3 cups a day.

Sinus Tea for Kiddos

YIELD: 3 CUPS

2 teaspoons dried rose hips

1 teaspoon dried oregano leaves

1 teaspoon dried peppermint leaves

1 teaspoon dried thyme leaves

3 cups boiling water

Combine the rose hips, oregano leaves, peppermint leaves, and thyme leaves in a bowl. Add the boiling water and steep for 30 minutes. Strain and discard the solids. Serve warm. Stored in a sealed glass jar in the refrigerator, Sinus Tea for Kiddos will keep for 48 hours.

DOSAGE: For children five years of age and older: ½ to 1 cup, 1 to 3 times a day.

Shower Soother

YIELD: ENOUGH FOR 1 USE

1 cup baking soda

½ cup citric acid

½ cup cornstarch

⅓ cup Epsom salts or coarse sea salt

1¾ tablespoons water

1½ tablespoons apricot, almond, or grapeseed oil

½ teaspoon eucalyptus, tea tree, or thyme essential oil

¼ teaspoon borax

Put the baking soda, citric acid, cornstarch, and Epsom salts in a mound in the bathtub or on floor of the shower. Combine the water, apricot oil, essential oil, and borax in a cup and mix well. Pour over the baking soda mixture.

APPLICATION INSTRUCTIONS: For children five years of age and older: Turn on the shower. Have the child stand in the shower and breathe the steam. If the smell is too overpowering, have the child sit elsewhere in the bathroom and breathe in the vapor.

Sinus Extract Blend

YIELD: 3 OUNCES

2 tablespoons goldenrod extract

1 tablespoon astragalus extract

1 tablespoon echinacea extract

1 tablespoon elder flower extract

1 tablespoon wild indigo extract

Combine all the ingredients in a glass dropper bottle. Stored in a cool, dry place, Sinus Extract Blend will keep for 2 years.

DOSAGE:

- For children six to ten years of age: 10 to 15 drops, 2 or 3 times a day.
- For children eleven to fifteen years of age: 20 to 25 drops, 2 or 3 times a day.
- For teens sixteen years of age and older: 25 to 40 drops, 2 or 3 times a day.

Sinus Headache Bath Salts YIELD: ENOUGH FOR 15 BATHS

2 to 3 cups Epsom salts

1 cup sea salt

⅓ cup dried peppermint leaves, crushed

⅓ cup dried spearmint leaves, crushed

40 drops peppermint essential oil

20 drops eucalyptus or rosemary essential oil

Combine the Epsom salts, sea salt, peppermint leaves, and spearmint leaves in a large bowl. Gradually add the essential oils and mix well. Stored in a tightly sealed container, Sinus Headache Bath Salts will keep for 1 year.

APPLICATION INSTRUCTIONS: For children six years of age and older: Add ¼ to ⅓ cup per bath. (Note: This can be somewhat messy. For easier cleanup, use a mesh strainer in the drain.)

Sinus Headache Pillow YIELD: 1 (10 X 4-INCH) PILLOW

½ cup whole flaxseeds

2 tablespoons dried spearmint leaves, crushed

2 tablespoons dried whole lavender buds

1 tablespoon dried eucalyptus leaves, crushed

1 tablespoon dried peppermint leaves, crushed

1 tablespoon dried rosemary leaves

2 (10 x 4-inch) pieces of fabric

Combine the flaxseeds, spearmint leaves, lavender buds, eucalyptus leaves, peppermint leaves, and rosemary leaves in a large bowl and mix well. Set aside.

Put the right sides of the fabric together and sew up three sides of the rectangle and almost all of the fourth side, leaving just enough space to insert the herbal mixture. Turn the rectangle right-side out and press it with an iron. Fill the bag with the herb mixture and sew it closed.

APPLICATION INSTRUCTIONS: For children four years of age and older: Place on the eyes for a soothing rest.

Sinus Mustard

½ cup whole brown or yellow mustard seeds

¼ cup brown sugar

1 teaspoon sea salt

1 teaspoon ground black or white pepper

1 teaspoon ground turmeric

1 clove garlic, crushed, or ½ to 1 tablespoon grated horseradish

⅞ cup apple cider vinegar

Put the mustard seeds, sugar, salt, pepper, turmeric, and garlic in a food processor and process until well combined. With the machine running, add the vinegar, 1 tablespoon at a time, through the cap opening in the lid, using just enough to form a coarse paste. Set aside for 20 minutes.

Transfer to a glass jar, seal, and refrigerate for 2 weeks before using. Stored in the refrigerator, Sinus Mustard will keep for 3 months.

NOTE: Children six years of age and younger should not use mustard medicinally; children four years of age and younger should not use horseradish medicinally.

APPLICATION INSTRUCTIONS: For children six years of age and older: Use as a condiment on food to help clear sinuses. Sometimes if the child just smells the mixture it will do the job.

Calendula Salve

YIELD: 6 TO 8 (4-ounce) SALVES

½ cup grated beeswax

2 cups calendula infused oil

1 teaspoon vitamin E oil

To make a salve, melt the beeswax in a small saucepan over medium-low heat. Stir in the infused oil and vitamin E oil. Pour into salve pots and set aside until firm. Stored in sealed salve pots at room temperature, Calendula Salve will keep for 1 year.

NOTE: Vitamin E oil is generally available in two strengths—32,000 IU and 45,000 IU. Either strength can be used in this recipe.

APPLICATION INSTRUCTIONS: For children two months of age and older: Apply as needed to the affected area.

Plantain Salve

YIELD: 6 TO 8 (4-ounce) SALVES

This salve is a useful remedy for many conditions, including abrasions, bug bites, cold sores, diaper rash, dry skin, eczema, inflammations, scrapes, stings, stretch marks, and superficial burns.

½ cup grated beeswax

2 cups infused plantain oil

1 teaspoon vitamin E oil

To make a salve, melt the beeswax in a small saucepan over medium-low heat. Stir in the infused oil and vitamin E oil. Pour into salve pots and set aside until firm. Stored in sealed salve pots at room temperature, Plantain Salve will keep for 6 months.

NOTE: Vitamin E oil is generally available in two strengths—32,000 IU and 45,000 IU. Either strength can be used in this recipe.

APPLICATION INSTRUCTIONS: For children two months and older: Apply as needed to the affected area.

Soothing Salve

1 cup fresh plantain leaves

1 cup fresh comfrey leaves

1 cup fresh St. John's wort flowers

1 cup fresh calendula flowers

Olive oil, enough to cover the herbs

1 cup grated beeswax

30 drops lavender or tea tree essential oil

Following the directions for making infused oil on page 177, prepare an infused oil using the plantain leaves, comfrey leaves, St. John's wort flowers, calendula flowers, and olive oil.

To make a salve, melt the beeswax in a small saucepan over medium-low heat. Stir in the infused oil and essential oil. Pour into salve pots and set aside until firm. Stored in sealed salve pots at room temperature, Soothing Salve will keep for 2 years.

APPLICATION INSTRUCTIONS: For children one year of age and older: Rub a small amount of the salve on raw rashes and on burns after they've cooled.

See also: **Comfrey Compress,** page 176

First-Aid Remedy, page 161

Goldenseal Salve, page 154

St. John's Wort Salve, page 164

Slippery Elm Cough Drops   YIELD: 20 TO 30 COUGH DROPS

2 cups water

¼ cup slippery elm bark powder

2 tablespoons honey, agave nectar, or other sweetener (optional)

1 drop peppermint, ginger, thyme, or fennel essential oil (optional)

Combine the water and slippery elm bark powder in a medium saucepan and bring to a simmer over medium-high heat, stirring gently to prevent clumping. Remove from the heat and let stand for 30 minutes. For a sweeter or more flavorful cough drop, add the optional honey and essential oil.

Stir the mixture until it is thick and pliable. Roll out on a flat surface to a thickness of about ⅛ inch or less. Cut into small circles or squares of equal size. (Try using a bottle cap or a wide pastry bag tip as a cutter.) Let dry at room temperature. Stored in a tin or other airtight container, Slippery Elm Cough Drops will keep for 3 to 6 months.

DOSAGE: For children six years of age (or younger if they are able to eat hard candy) and older: 2 to 5 cough drops a day.

Comfrey Compress   YIELD: ENOUGH FOR 2 TO 3 COMPRESSES

Do not use this compress on puncture wounds, scrapes, or broken skin.

2 large fresh comfrey leaves, chopped

2 cups boiling water

Put the comfrey leaves in a bowl. Add the boiling water and steep until completely cool.

APPLICATION INSTRUCTIONS: For children three years of age and older: Saturate a cloth with the tea and apply to the affected area 3 times, 2 times a day.

Simple Clove Tea

YIELD: 4 CUPS

This tea is too strongly flavored for babies and toddlers, so do not use it for children younger than two years of age. To make the tea more palatable, mix it with juice.

4 cups water   1 teaspoon whole cloves

Put the water and cloves in a medium saucepan over medium heat and bring to a simmer. Simmer for 20 minutes. Remove from the heat and steep for 20 minutes. Strain and discard the cloves. Serve warm. Stored in a covered container in the refrigerator, Simple Clove Tea will keep for 48 hours.

NOTE: Do not give more than the recommended dose. Too great a quantity of cloves can irritate the stomach, so more is not better in this case.

DOSAGE:

- For children two to four years of age: 1 tablespoon, 2 to 3 times a day.
- For children five to six years of age: 2 tablespoons, 2 to 3 times a day.
- For children seven to eight years of age: ½ cup, 2 to 3 times a day.
- For children nine years of age and older: ½ to 1 cup, 2 to 3 times a day.

Tummy Glycerite

YIELD: VARIES WITH QUANTITY MADE

1 part fresh peppermint leaves

1 part fresh lemon balm

1 part coarsely chopped fresh ginger

Vegetable glycerin

Following the directions for making extracts on page 118, prepare an extract using equal amounts of peppermint, lemon balm, and ginger root in vegetable glycerin. Stored in a glass jar in the refrigerator, Tummy Glycerite will keep for 3 to 8 months.

DOSAGE:

- For children one to three years of age: 10 to 15 drops, 2 to 3 times a day.
- For children four to six years of age: 15 to 20 drops, 2 to 3 times a day.
- For children seven to ten years of age: 20 to 30 drops, 2 to 3 times a day.
- For children eleven to fifteen years of age: 30 to 40 drops, 2 to 3 times a day.

See also: **Rose Hips Tea,** page 141

Baby Gumming Rub   YIELD: ABOUT 6 TABLESPOONS

This rub often supplies instant relief for a cranky, teething baby.

> 1 cup water
> 1 teaspoon whole cloves
> 2 tablespoons vegetable glycerin

Bring the water to a boil in a small saucepan over medium-high heat. Add the cloves. Decrease the heat to medium-low and simmer for 20 minutes. Remove from the heat and cool to room temperature. Strain and discard the cloves.

Combine ¼ cup of the strained liquid with the vegetable glycerin in a small glass jar or storage container. (The remaining liquid may be frozen in an ice cube tray for future use.) Cover tightly. Stored in a sealed container in the refrigerator, Baby Gumming Rub will keep for 2 to 6 months.

APPLICATION INSTRUCTIONS: For babies four months of age and older: Pour a drop on your finger and rub it on the baby's gums.

Peppermint Rub   YIELD: 2 TABLESPOONS

Glycerin tastes sweet, which makes this remedy appealing to children.

> 2 tablespoons vegetable oil or vegetable glycerin
> 1 drop peppermint essential oil

Combine the ingredients in a small, clean, dry jar. Cover and shake to combine. Stored in a sealed glass jar in the refrigerator, Peppermint Rub will keep for 2 to 6 months.

APPLICATION INSTRUCTIONS: For babies four months of age and older: Apply just a tiny dab to the affected gum 2 to 3 times a day.

Slippery Elm Paste

¼ cup cold water or juice
1½ teaspoons slippery elm bark powder

Combine the water and slippery elm bark powder in a small cup or bowl and stir to make a paste. Stored in a sealed glass jar in the refrigerator, Slippery Elm Paste will keep for 48 hours.

APPLICATION INSTRUCTIONS: For babies four months of age and older: Apply a dab to the affected gum as needed, or apply 4 to 5 times a day.

WHOOPING COUGH (PERTUSSIS)

Cough-Stop Tea

YIELD: 3 CUPS

This is a good nighttime tea.

1 tablespoon fresh thyme, or 2 teaspoons dried
1 tablespoon fresh elecampane root, or 2 teaspoons dried
1 tablespoon fresh red clover flowers, or 2 teaspoons dried
3 cups water

Combine the thyme, elecampane root, and red clover flowers in a small bowl. Bring the water to a boil in a medium saucepan. Stir in the herb mixture and remove from the heat. Steep for 20 minutes. Strain and discard the herbs. Serve warm. Stored in a sealed glass jar in the refrigerator, Cough-Stop Tea will keep for 48 hours.

DOSAGE: For children four years of age and older: ½ cup before bedtime, but no more than 1 cup of tea per 24-hour period. Do not administer during a coughing fit.

Super-Cough Tea

This is a good tea to use for daytime coughs.

- 5 cups water
- 3 cinnamon sticks
- 2 (3-inch) pieces licorice root, or ¼ cup chopped licorice root
- 4 teaspoons dried thyme

Bring the water to a simmer in a medium saucepan over medium heat. Add the cinnamon sticks and licorice root and simmer for 20 minutes. Remove from the heat and add the thyme. Steep for 15 to 20 minutes. Strain and discard the herbs. Serve warm.

DOSAGE:

- For babies six months to two years of age: Seek medical advice.
- For children two to three years of age: 3 teaspoons, 2 to 3 times a day.
- For children four years of age and older: 1 cup, 3 times a day.

Three Fun Herb Gardens

hese gardens, which are quite different from each other, can easily be modified to fit your needs. Growing an herb garden can be great fun, a good learning experience for children and parents, and a way to spend time together in nature.

A SACRED GARDEN

his garden is built in and around four concentric stone circles representing the four elements: earth, wind, fire, and water. The diameter of the entire garden is thirty feet.

Gather together thirty-six rocks: twleve small (about the size of your fist), twelve medium (about the size of your head), and twelve very large (about knee height). Outline a circle with a diameter equal to your height and place the twelve smallest stones around the circle like numbers around a clock face.

Lie with your feet at one rock and your head away from the first circle of stones to mark the perimeter of the second circle. Use the medium stones to mark the second circle as you did the first. Repeat with the largest stones for the largest circle. You now have four planting zones: inside the first circle of stones, outside the first circle, outside the second circle, and outside the third circle. These planting zones represent the four elements of matter.

I recommend the following plants to represent each realm in this garden because of their medicinal capabilities, their associations with certain bodily systems, and the needs they fill. Of course, you must substitute plants that are important to you. Your sacred garden should represent what is sacred to *you*.

The realm of earth is represented in the circle at the center of the garden. In this area, plant:

lady's mantle (*Alchemilla vulgaris*)
lady's slipper (*Cypripedium acaule*)
pennyroyal (*Mentha pulegium*)
rue (*Ruta graveolens*)
skullcap (*Scutellaria lateriflora*)
tansy (*Tanacetum vulgare*)
valerian (*Valeriana officinalis*)
wormwood (*Artemisia absinthium*)

The realm of water lies between the perimeters of the first and second circles. In this area, plant:

black willow (*Salix nigra*)
burdock (*Arctium lappa*)
catnip (*Nepeta cataria*)
chickweed (*Stellaria media*)
cleavers (*Galium aparine*)
echinacea (*Echinacea purpurea*)
hops (*Humulus lupulus*)
horsetail (*Equisetum arvense*)
rosemary (*Rosmarinus officinalis*)
violet (*Viola odorata*)

The realm of air lies between the second and third circles. In this area, plant:

calendula (*Calendula officinalis*)
chamomile (*Matricaria recutita*)
hyssop (*Hyssopus officinalis*)
lavender (*Lavandula angustifolia*)
peppermint (*Mentha piperita*)
spearmint (*Mentha spicata*)
vervain (*Verbena officinalis*)
yarrow (*Achillea millefolium*)

The realm of fire lies outside the third stone circle. In this area, plant:

aloe vera (Aloe *barbadensis*)

buckthorn (*Rhamnus cathartica*)

butterfly weed (*Asclepias tuberosa*)

fireweed (*Erechtites hieracifolia*)

habanero (*Capsicum chinense*)

jalapeño (*Capsicum annuum*)

St. John's wort (*Hypericum perforatum*)

white oak (*Quercus alba*)

witch hazel (*Hamamelis virginiana*)

SEASONAL GARDENS

Plants have what I call "spiritual seasons." In other words, they contain the essence of certain seasons.

When planted at a school, a seasonal garden can be a great project for students and teachers. It is fun, multidimensional, textural, and full of color. It also attracts bees and butterflies, lending itself to lessons not only about plants but also about animals, pollination, the environment, and the preservation of nature. The following garden is much like one I designed for the Nature School in Greenville, New Hampshire.

Spring

anise (*Pimpinella anisum*)

basil (*Ocimum basilicum*)

chervil (*Anthriscus cerefolium*)

coltsfoot (*Tussilago farfara*)

dandelion (*Taraxacum officinale*)

ginger *(Zingiber officinale)*

peppermint (*Mentha piperita*)

sage (*Salvia officinalis*)

spearmint (*Mentha spicata*)

Summer

angelica (*Angelica archangelica*)

bee balm (*Monarda didyma* or *Monarda fistulosa*)

borage (*Borago officinalis*)

elder (*Sambucus nigra*)

marshmallow (*Althaea officinalis*)

plantain (*Plantago major*)

red clover (*Trifolium pratense*)

rue (*Ruta graveolens*)

Autumn

burdock (*Arctium lappa*)

calendula (*Calendula officinalis*)

elecampane (*Inula helenium*)

St. John's wort (*Hypericum perforatum*)

yarrow (*Achillea millefolium*)

Winter

echinacea (*Echinacea purpurea*)

corn (*Zea mays*)

fenugreek (*Trigonella foenum-graecum*)

costmary (*Tanacetum balsamita*)

chickweed (*Stellaria media*)

PURPOSE PATCHES

Purpose patches are small gardens containing plants that have a single medical, therapeutic, or synergistic purpose. You can plant several of these patches, depending on your family's needs.

Children's Garden

Choose every plant you could possibly need to treat common childhood illnesses:

aloe vera (*Aloe barbadensis*)

bilberry (*Vaccinium myrtillus*)

calendula (*Calendula officinalis*)

mullein (*Verbascum thapsus*)

peppermint (*Mentha piperita*)

plantain (*Plantago major*)

roses (*Rosa canina* and *R. majalis*)

sage (*Salvia officinalis*)

thyme (*Thymus vulgaris*)

Digestive Patch

anise (*Pimpinella anisum*)

caraway (*Carum carvi*)

catnip (*Nepeta cataria*)

chamomile (*Matricaria recutita*)

fennel (*Foeniculum vulgare*)

lemon balm (*Melissa officinalis*)

peppermint (*Mentha piperita*)

Liver Patch

anise (*Pimpinella anisum*)

burdock (*Arctium lappa*)

dandelion (*Taraxacum officinale*)

stinging nettle (*Urtica dioica*)

peppermint (*Mentha piperita*)

rosemary (*Rosmarinus officinalis*)

PMS Patch

This garden is especially nice when planted in a spiral.

lady's mantle (*Alchemilla vulgaris*)
motherwort (*Leonurus cardiaca*)
red raspberry (*Rubus idaeus*)
sweet cicely (*Myrrhis odorata*)
valerian (*Valeriana officinalis*)

Tone and Nourish the Blood Patch

comfrey (*Symphytum officinale*)
dandelion (*Taraxacum officinale*)
peppermint (*Mentha piperita*)
primrose (*Primula vulgaris*)
stinging nettle (*Urtica dioica*)
yarrow (*Achillea millefolium*)

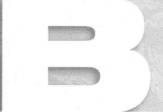

Herbs as Nutritional Supplements

In addition to having medicinal properties, herbs can be rich in nutrients. The following herbs are great sources of vitamins and minerals. They can easily be grown or foraged, and most are inexpensive additions to a more healthful diet. In this age of "superfoods," we can find many right in our own herb gardens, and at a fraction of the cost of the latest trend.

Get creative and add herbs to your family's foods. Juice them with fruits and vegetables. Eat them raw or in an extract, an infusion, or a decoction. Add a teaspoonful to a tablespoonful to kids' foods and drinks for a boost of nutrition.

Vitamin A: *Alfalfa, dandelion, garlic*

Prepare an alfalfa-rich infusion. Add dandelion or garlic to salads, sauces, and soups.

Vitamin C: *Alfalfa, dandelion, garlic, papaya, rose hips, horseradish, yellow dock*

Use alfalfa as an infusion, added to salad dressings, smoothies, and soups. Add garlic and horseradish to salads, soups, and spreads. Use the papaya and rose hips in sorbets and smoothies. (**Note:** Horseradish should not be given to children four years of age and younger.)

Vitamin E: *Alfalfa, dandelion, dong quai (Angelica sinensis), red raspberry, rose hips, watercress*

Add rose hips and raspberries to salads, salad dressings, and smoothies. Use dandelion and watercress in salads, sandwiches, and soups.

Calcium: *Alfalfa, blue cohosh (Caulophyllum thalictroides), chamomile, chlorophyll, dandelion, irish moss (Sagina subulata), rose hips, yarrow, yellow dock*

Iron: *Alfalfa, burdock, blue cohosh, chlorophyll, dandelion, mullein, parsley*

Use dandelion greens in salads and smoothies. Add a handful of parsley to just about anything.

glossary

Antioxidant. Antioxidants protect cells from the effects of free radicals. Free radicals are substances (such as cigarette smoke) that cause healthy cells to oxidize, or age.

Berberine. Berberine is a compound in goldenseal that may displace bilirubin in babies.

Bioflavonoids. Bioflavonoids are the natural pigments in fruits and vegetables that help prevent cellular damage caused by free radicals.

Chilblains. Chilblains is a condition occurs in cold weather and causes itching and burning. It is marked by redness and swelling of the ears, fingers, nose, and toes. Cracking of the skin and ulceration sometimes occur.

Diffusion. An essential oil is diffused so that its scent and potential therapeutic value fill a room or an area. This is usually done with a diffuser, blowing air, or heat.

Linalol. Linalol is an essential oil derived from thyme.

Materia medica. A materia medica is a list of remedies and how they can be used.

Nutritional yeast. An inactive yeast, similar to but not the same as brewer's yeast, nutritional yeast is high in B vitamins and is used in cooking as a nutritional supplement. It is available in powder form and in yellow flakes.

suppliers

HERBS AND HERB PLANTS

Adaptations
808-328-9044

Permaculture-grown tropical plants, including ginger, gotu kola, kava, and passionflower.

Attar Herbs & Spices
www.attarherbs.com

Frontier Natural Products Co-op
www.frontiercoop.com

Garden Medicinals
www.gardenmedicinals.com

Horizon Herbs
www.horizonherbs.com

Longevity Herb Company
http://business.gorge.net/longevity

Medicinal Herb Plants
www.medicinalherbplants.com

Mountain Rose Herbs
www.mountainroseherbs.com

Mt. Eden Greenhouse
502-738-5502

Awesome plant collection that's sure to have what you want.

Nature's Cathedral
www.naturescathedral.com

Echinacea, goldenseal, and other cultivated herbs.

Pacific Botanicals
www.pacificbotanicals.com

High-quality organic and wildcrafted herbs. Will deliver fresh plants.

Richters Herbs
www.richters.com

Southern Virginia Herbals
www.gardenmedicinals.com/pages/va_sources.html

Organic herbs from the East and Southeast.

CHINESE HERBS

Spring Wind Herbs
www.springwind.com

Starwest Botanicals
www.starwest-botanicals.com

HERB SEEDS

Abundant Life Seeds
www.abundantlifeseeds.com

Bountiful Gardens
www.bountifulgardens.org

Fedco Seeds
www.fedcoseeds.com

Harris Seeds
www.harrisseeds.com

High Mowing Organic Seeds
www.highmowingseeds.com

Johnny's Selected Seeds
www.johnnyseeds.com

Seed Savers Exchange
www.seedsavers.org

Seeds From Italy
www.growitalian.com

Seeds of Change
www.seedsofchange.com

Territorial Seed Company
www.territorialseed.com

BOTTLES AND CONTAINERS

Acme Vial & Glass Company, Inc.
www.acmevial.com

Berlin Packaging
www.berlinpackaging.com

BASCO
www.bascousa.com

Cape Bottle Company
www.netbottle.com

Cleveland Bottle & Supply Co.
www.clevelandbottle.com

E. D. Luce Packaging
www.essentialsupplies.com

General Bottle Supply
www.bottlesetc.com

**Industrial Container
and Supply Company**
www.industrialcontainer.com

Mid-Continent AgriMarketing, Inc.
800-547-1392
Also supplies beeswax, dyes, jars, molds, and scents.

Packaging West, Inc.
www.tricorbraun.com
Also supplies droppers, jars, salves, and tins.

SKS Bottle & Packaging, Inc.
www.sks-bottle.com

Sunburst Bottle Company
www.sunburstbottle.com

OILS, BEESWAX, AND TEABAGS

Attar Herbs and Spices
www.attarherbs.com

**Bramble Berry
Soap Making Supplies**
www.brambleberry.com

Columbus Foods
www.soaperschoice.com

From Nature with Love
www.fromnaturewithlove.com

Liberty Natural Products, Inc.
www.libertynatural.com

Rainbow Meadow, Inc.
www.rainbowmeadow.com

Western Plastics Corp.
www.uscontainer.com

SALVES AND SOAPS

Bean Tree Soaps
www.beantreesoap.com

Botanical Earth
www.botanicalearth.com

Dreamseeds Organics
http://hyenacart.com/dreamseeds

Great Cape Herbs
www.greatcape.com

Green Goddess Garden
www.masterwort.com

Kerry's Herbals
www.kerrysherbals.com

Maine Coast Herbals
www.maineherbs.com

Motherlove Herbal Company
www.motherlove.com

Mountain Rose Herbs
www.mountainroseherbs.com

Purple Shutter Herbs
www.purpleshutter.com

Red Moon Herbs
www.redmoonherbs.com

San Francisco Herb Co.
www.sfherb.com

Stony Mountain Botanicals
www.wildroots.com

WiseWays Herbals
www.wiseways.com

TEAPOTS

Bodum Teapots
www.bodum.com

YiXing Teapots
www.yixing.com

VINEGAR

Bragg Live Foods
www.bragg.com

Sonoma Vinegar Works
www.sonomavinegarworks.com

TINS

Jean's Greens
www.jeansgreens.com

associations and schools

HERB ASSOCIATIONS

American Herb Association
www.ahaherb.com

American Herbalists Guild
www.americanherbalistguild.com

Herb Research Foundation
www.herbs.org

**National Association
for Holistic Aromatherapy**
www.naha.org

United Plant Savers
www.unitedplantsavers.org

HERBALISM SCHOOLS

Bastyr University
www.bastyr.edu

**East West School
of Planetary Herbology**
www.planetherbs.com

Heart of Herbs Herbal School
www.heartofherbs.com
*The author, Demetria Clark,
is founder and director.*

Herbal Therapeutics
www.herbaltherapeutics.net

Sage Mountain
www.sagemt.com

Wise Woman Center
www.susunweed.com

recommended reading

For more information about herbal remedies for children:

Block, M. A. *No More Antibiotics: Preventing and Treating Ear and Respiratory Infections the Natural Way.* New York: Kensington, 2000.

Bove, M. *Encyclopedia of Natural Healing for Children and Infants.* Chicago: Keats Publishing, 2001.

Galland, L. *Power Healing: Use the New Integrated Medicine to Cure Yourself.* New York: Random House, 1998.

Gladstar, R. *Herbal Remedies for Children's Health.* North Adams, MA: Storey Publishing, 1999.

———. *Rosemary Gladstar's Family Herbal: A Guide to Living Life with Energy, Health, and Vitality.* North Adams, MA: Storey Publishing, 2001.

Levy, J. *Nature's Children: A Guide to Organic Foods and Herbal Remedies for Children.* Woodstock, NY: Ash Tree Publishing, 1996.

McIntyre, A. *Herbal for Mother and Child.* London: Thorsons, 2003.

Mendelsohn, R. S. *How to Raise a Healthy Child In Spite of Your Doctor.* New York: Ballantine, 1987.

Romm, A. J. *Naturally Healthy Babies and Children: A Commonsense Guide to Herbal Remedies, Nutrition, and Health.* Berkeley, CA: Celestial Arts, 2004.

Schmidt, M. A., and D. Rapp. *Healing Childhood Ear Infections: Prevention, Home Care, and Alternative Treatment.* Berkeley, CA: North Atlantic Books, 1996.

Tierra, L. *Kid's Herbal Book.* San Francisco: Robert D. Reed Publishers, 2000.

White, L. B., and S. Mavor. *Kids, Herbs, and Health: A Parent's Guide to Natural Remedies.* Loveland, CO: Interweave Press, 1999.

Zand, J. *Smart Medicine for a Healthier Child: A Practical A-to-Z Reference to Natural and Conventional Treatments for Infants and Children.* New York: Avery Publishing, 1994.

For more information about making herbal and aromatherapy remedies:

Arnould-Taylor, W. E. *A Textbook of Holistic Aromatherapy: The Use of Essential Oils Treatments*. Philadelphia, PA: Trans-Atlantic Publications, 1992.

Cech, R. *Making Plant Medicine*. Williams, OR: Horizon Herbs, 2000.

Close, B. *Aromatherapy: The A–Z Guide to Healing with Essential Oils*. New York: Dell, 1997.

Dodt, C., and D. Balmuth. *Essential Oils Book: Creating Personal Blends for Mind and Body*. North Adams, MA: Storey Publishing, 1996.

Fischer-Rizzi, S. *Complete Aromatherapy Handbook: Essential Oils for Radiant Health*. New York: Sterling, 1991.

Gattefosse, R., and R. Tisserand. *Gattefosse's Aromatherapy: The First Book on Aromatherapy*. London: Random House, 2004.

Gladstar, R. *Rosemary Gladstar's Herbal Recipes for Vibrant Health: 175 Teas, Tonics, Oils, Salves, Tinctures, and Other Natural Remedies for the Entire Family*. North Adams, MA: Storey Publishing, 2008.

Grace, U. *Aromatherapy for Practitioners*. London: C. W. Daniel, 2009.

Green, J. *Herbal Medicine Maker's Handbook: A Home Manual*. Freedom, CA: Crossing Press, 2000.

Grieve, M. *Modern Herbal (Volume 1, A–H)* and *A Modern Herbal (Volume 2, H–Z)*. Whitefish, MT: Kessinger, 2006.

Hoffman, D. *Herbal Handbook: A User's Guide to Medical Herbalism*. Rochester, VT: Healing Arts Press, 1998.

Mabey, R., and M. McIntyre. *New Age Herbalist: How to Use Herbs for Healing, Nutrition, Body Care, and Relaxation*. New York: Fireside, 1988.

Price, S. *Aromatherapy for Common Ailments*. New York: Fireside, 1991.

———. *Practical Aromatherapy*. London: Thorsons, 2000.

Rose, J. *Aromatherapy Book*. Berkeley, CA: North Atlantic Books, 1993.

———. *Herbs and Things: Jeanne Rose's Herbal*. San Francisco: Last Gasp, 2001.

———. *World of Aromatherapy: An Anthology of Aromatic History, Ideas, Concepts and Case Histories*. Berkeley, CA: Frog Ltd., 1996.

Ryman, D. *Aromatherapy Handbook*. London: C. W. Daniel, 2004.

———. *Aromatherapy: The Complete Guide to Plant and Flower Essences for Health and Beauty*. New York: Bantam, 1993.

Schiller, C., D. Schiller, and J. Schiller. *Aromatherapy Oils: A Complete Guide*. New York: Sterling, 1996.

Schnaubelt, K. *Advanced Aromatherapy*. Rochester, VT: Healing Arts Press, 1995.

———. *Medical Aromatherapy*. Berkeley, CA: Frog Ltd., 1999.

Tisserand, M. *Aromatherapy for Women: A Practical Guide to Essential Oils for Health and Beauty*. Rochester, VT: Healing Arts Press, 1988.

Tisserand, R. *Aromatherapy*. London: C. W. Daniel, 2004.

Tisserand, R., and T. Balacs. *Essential Oil Safety*. London: Churchill Livingstone, 1995.

Wildwood, C. *Encyclopedia of Aromatherapy*. Rochester, VT: Healing Arts Press, 1996.

Worwood, V. A. *Complete Book of Essential Oils and Aromatherapy*. Novato, CA: New World Library, 1991.

Valnet, J., and R. Tisserand. *Practice of Aromatherapy: A Classic Compendium of Plant Medicines and Their Healing Properties*. Rochester, VT: Healing Arts Press, 1982.

For more information about growing your own herbs:

Brennan, G. *Little Herb Gardens: Simple Secrets for Glorious Gardens Indoors and Out*. San Francisco: Chronicle Books, 2004.

Cech, R. *Growing At-Risk Medicinal Herbs, Cultivation, Conservation, and Ecology*. Williams, OR: Horizon Herbs, 2002.

De La Tour, S. *Herbalist's Garden: A Guided Tour of 10 Exceptional Herb Gardens, The People Who Grow Them and the Plants That Inspire Them*. North Adams, MA: Storey Publishing, 2001.

Hirsch, D. *Moosewood Restaurant Kitchen Garden*. Berkeley, CA: Ten Speed Press, 2005.

Kavasch, E. B. *Medicine Wheel Garden: Creating Sacred Space for Healing, Celebration, and Tranquility*. New York: Bantam, 2002.

McIntyre, A. *Good Health Garden: Growing and Using Healing Foods*. New York: Reader's Digest, 1998.

Smith, M. *Your Backyard Herb Garden: A Gardener's Guide to Growing over 50 Herbs Plus How to Use Them in Cooking, Crafts, Companion Planting, and More*. Emmaus, PA: Rodale, 1999.

Sombke, L. *Beautiful Easy Herbs: How to Get the Most from Herbs—In Your Garden and in Your Home*. Emmaus, PA: Rodale, 2000.

Sturdivant, L., and T. Blakley. *The Bootstrap Guide to Medicinal Herbs in the Garden, Field, and Marketplace*. Friday Harbor, WA: San Juan Naturals, 1998.

For more information about harvesting and preserving herbs:

Belt, T. E. *Preserving Winemaking Ingredients: How to "Put Down" Your Flowers. Herbs, Fruits and Vegetables by Drying, Deep-Freezing, Bottling or Chemical Preservation, and How to Make a Whole Range of Unusual Syrups, Jams and Jellies.* Amateur Winemaker, 1969.

Chioffi, N. *Keeping the Harvest: Preserving Your Fruits, Vegetables, and Herbs.* North Adams, MA: Storey Publishing, 1991.

Duke, J. A., and S. Foster. *Field Guide to Medicinal Plants and Herbs of Eastern and Central North America.* New York: Houghton Mifflin Harcourt, 1999.

Hopping, J. W. *Pioneer Lady's Country Kitchen: A Seasonal Treasury of Time-Honored American Recipes.* New York: Villard Books, 1992.

Romanné-James, C. *Herb-Lore for Housewives.* Farmington Hills, MI: Gale Research, 1998.

Simmons, A. G. *Herbs Are Forever: Caprilands' Guide to Growing and Preserving.* New York: BDD Promotional Books, 1992.

For more information about herb crafting:

Flanders, A. *Aromatics: Potpourris, Oils, and Scented Delights to Enhance Your Home and Heal Your Spirit.* New York: Clarkson Potter, 1995.

Kelly, R. "Make 22 Herbal Gifts for the Holidays." *Storey Publishing Bulletin*, 1995; A-149.

Long, J. *Making Herbal Dream Pillows: Secret Blends for Pleasant Dreams.* North Adams, MA: Storey Books, 2003.

Nadeau, A. *Making and Selling Herbal Crafts: Tips, Techniques, Projects.* New York: Sterling, 1996.

Newdick, J. *At Home With Herbs.* North Adams, MA: Storey Books, 1994.

Shaudys, P. *Herbal Treasures: Inspiring Month-By-Month Projects for Gardening, Cooking, and Crafts.* North Adams, MA: Storey Books, 1992.

bibliography

Beers, M. H. *The Merck Manual of Medical Information, Second Home Edition*. Whitehouse Station, NJ: Merck Research Laboratories, 2003.

Blumenthal M., W. R. Busse, A. Goldberg, J. Gruenwald, T. Hall, C. W. Riggins, and R. S. Rister, eds. S. Klein and R. S. Rister, trans. *The Complete German Commission E Monographs*. Austin, TX: American Botanical Council, 1998.

Blumenthal M., A. Goldberg, and J. Brinckmann. *Herbal Medicine: The Expanded Commission E Monographs*. Newton, MA: Integrative Medicine Communications, 2000.

Diener, H. C., V. W. Rahlfs, and U. Danesch. "The First Placebo-Controlled Trial of a Special Butterbur Root Extract for the Prevention of Migraine: Reanalysis of Efficacy Criteria." *Eur Neurol,* 2004;51(2): 89–97.

Foda M., P. F. Middlebrook, C. T. Gatfield, et al. "Efficacy of Cranberry in Prevention of Urinary Tract Infection in a Susceptible Pediatric Population." *Canadian J Urol,* 1991;2(1): 98–102.

Gibson L., L. Pike, and J. Kilbourne. "Effectiveness of Cranberry Juice in Preventing Urinary Tract Infections in Long-Term Care Facility Patients." *J Naturopath Med,* 1991;2(1): 45–47.

Glass, R. I., A. M. Svennerholm, B. J. Stoll, M. R. Khan, K. Hossain, and J. Holmgren. "Protection Against Cholera in Breast-Fed Children by Antibodies in Breast Milk." *N Eng J Med,* 1983;308:1389–1392.

Grossman, W., and H. Schmidramsl. "An Extract of *Petasites hybridus* is Effective in the Prophylaxis of Migraine." *Altern Med Rev,* 2001;6(3): 303–310.

Hirsch, L. "Common Menstrual Problems." www.kidshealth.org.

Hoffmann, D. *The New Holistic Herbal, Second Edition*. Rockport, MA: Element, 1990.

Lipkin, A. "Otitis Media—Chronic." Medline Plus. www.nlm.nih.gov.

Lipton, R. B., H. Gobel, K. M. Einhaupl, et al. "*Petasites hybridus* Root (Butterbur) is an Effective Preventive Treatment for Migraine." *Neurology,* 2004;63(12): 2240–44.

López-Alarcón, M., A. Fajardo. "Breast-Feeding Lowers the Frequency and Duration of Acute Respiratory Infection and Diarrhea in Infants Under Six Months of Age." *The Journal of Nutrition,* 1997;127:436–443.

Mills, S., and K. Bone. 2000. "Current Western Applications of Astragalus Are Primarily for Restoring and Strengthening the Immune Response, Enhancing Cardiovascular Function, and Increasing Vitality." *Principles and Practice of Phytotherapy,* 2003;273–279.

Newman, J. "How Breast Milk Protects Newborns." www.pregnancy.org.

Nostro, A., M. Cannatelli, G. Crisafi, and V. Alonzo. "The Effect of Nepeta Cataria Extract on Adherence and Enzyme Production of *Staphylococcus aureus.*" *Int J Antimicrob Agents,* 2001;18:583–585.

"Pertussis." www.wikipedia.com.

Ruiz, P., J. J. Calva, L. K. Pickering, Y. Lopez Vidal, P. Volkow, H. Pezzarossi, and M. S. West. "Protection of Breast-Fed Infants Against Campylobacter Diarrhea by Antibodies in Human Milk. *J Pediatr,* 1990;116: 707–713.

Saritas, Y., S. H. von Reuss, and W. A. Konig. "Sesquiterpene Constituents in *Petasites hybridus.*" *Phytochemistry,* 2002;59(8): 795–803.

Sarrell E. M., A. Mandelberg, and H. A. Cohen. "Efficacy of Naturopathic Extracts in the Management of Ear Pain Associated with Acute Otitis Media." *Arch Pediatr Adolesc Med,* 2001;155:796–799.

Science Daily. "Ginger May Combat Deadly Infant Diarrhea in Developing World." Oct. 4, 2007. www.sciencedaily.com/releases/2007/10/071001092216.htm.

Sears, J. "Ear Infections." www.askdrsears.com.

Sigerist, H. E. *A History of Medicine, Volume One.* New York: Oxford University, 1951.

Thomet, O. A., H. U. Simon. "Petasins in the Treatment of Allergic Diseases: Results of Preclinical and Clinical Studies." *Int Arch Allergy Immunol,* 2002;129(2): 108–12.

Thomet, O. A., U. N. Wiesmann, A. Schapowal, et al. "Role of Petasin in the Potential Anti-inflammatory Activity of a Plant Extract of *Petasites hybridus.*" *Biochem Pharmacol,* 2001;61(8): 1041–1047.

Weiss, R. F. *Herbal Medicine.* Beaconsfield: Arcanum, 1991.

Zakay-Rones, Z., E. Thom, T. Wollan, and J. Wadstein. "Randomized Study of the Efficacy and Safety of Oral Elderberry Extract in the Treatment of Influenza A and B Virus Infections." *J Int Med Res.* 2004;32(2): 132–140.

index

American Herbalist Guild, 18
American Medical Association (AMA), 20
anaphylaxis, mistletoe and, caution about, 61
androgens, 97
anemia: heavy periods and, 101, 102; treatments for, 2, 47, 50
Anethum graveolens (dill). *See* dill *(Anethum graveolens)*
angelica *(Angelica archangelica)*, 28; avoiding in sunshine, in essential oil form, 122; candied, 112; in garden, 184; as treatment, for dysmenorrhea (painful period), 100
Angelica archangelica (angelica). *See* angelica *(Angelica archangelica)*
Aniba roseaeodora (rosewood), 51, 98
anise *(Pimpinella anisum)*, 28; as essential oil, cautions about, 121, 122; in gardens, 183, 185; harvesting, *108*
ankle swelling, yarrow for treating, 58
annual herbs, 106, *108*
anodynes/analgesics, 25, 45
anorexia nervosa, burdock and, 31
Anthriscus cerefolium (chervil), in garden, 183
antibacterials/bactericides, 25; astragalus, 29; catnip, 32; cinnamon, 34; cloves, 35; goldenseal, 89; helichrysum, 40; horseradish, 42; rose petals, 50; thyme, 55, 92; usnea, 56
antibiotics: acne and, 96; **Anti-Gel,** 91, 158–159; diarrhea and, 82; for ear infections, 84; specific: bergamot, 30; breast milk, 78; eucalyptus, 79; garlic, 71, 84; lavender, 43; mullein, 84; pepper-

mint, 79; thrush and, 95; whooping cough and, 92
antidepressants, St. John's wort and, 53, 65
antifungals: black walnut, 30; catnip, 32; helichrysum, 41; tea tree, 54; thuja, 55
Anti-Gel, 91, 158–159
anti-inflammatories, 25; arnica, 29; astragalus, 29; calendula, 31; chamomile, 33; fennel, 39; licorice, 43, 92; meadowsweet, 44; potato, 77; red clover, 49; red raspberry leaf, 50; rose petals, 50; sage/red sage, 51; St. John's wort, 52; white oak bark, 56; yarrow, 58
antimicrobials, 26; anise, 28; echinacea, 36; garlic, 39; myrrh, 45; oregano, 46; thyme, 55
antioxidants, 189; in herbs: alfalfa, 27; astragalus, 29; hibiscus, 41; oregano, 46; rose petals, 50; sage/red sage, 51
antiseptics, 26; bergamot, 30; cinnamon, 34; elecampane, 37; frankincense, 38; horehound, 41; oregano, 46; tea tree, 54; thyme, 55; wild indigo, 57
antispasmodics, 26; anise, 28; bergamot, 30; cinnamon, 34; cloves, 35; fennel, 38; garlic, 39; mullein, 45; passionflower, 47; red clover, 49; rue, 51; sundew, 54, 92; thyme, 55, 92; wild cherry bark, 57; yarrow, 58, 59
antitussives, 54, 57, 92
antivirals: astragalus, 29; echinacea, 36; helichrysum, 41; lemon balm, 43; licorice, 43; oregano, 71; ravensara, 49
anxiety: cautions about, 59, 61; treatments for: nerv-

ines, 27; ***Rose Hips Tea,*** 141, 178; sedatives, 27; specific herbs: bergamot, 30; catnip, 32; chickweed, 33; clary sage, 34; ephedra, 59; frankincense, 38; goldenseal, 61; herbal teas, 72; lavender, 43; lemon balm, 43; motherwort, 44; passionflower, 47; peppermint, 48; rue, 51; skullcap, 51; St. John's wort, 53, 65; valerian, 72
Appalachia, 20, 22
appetite: herbs for stimulating: alfalfa, 27; angelica, 28; bergamot, 30; boneset, 31; burdock, 31; caraway, 32; fennel, 38; hibiscus, 41; peppermint, 48; lack of: chicken pox and, 70; constipation and, 78; ear infections and, 84; roseola and, 92
apricot kernel oil: as carrier oil, 67, 101, 121; in salves, 124
Aralia racemosa (spikenard), 62
Arctium lappa (burdock). *See* burdock *(Arctium lappa)*
Armoracia rusticana (horseradish). *See* horseradish *(Armoracia rusticana)*
arnica *(Arnica montana)*, 28–29; ***Arnica Compress, Plaintain-,*** 68, 136; cautions about, 59, 136; as treatment: for bruises, 65; for muscle aches and pains, 65, 91; for sprains, 94
Arnica montana (arnica). *See* arnica *(Arnica montana)*
aromatherapy, 122–123; author's study of, 3; for dysmenorrhea, 100; essential oils and, 120, 122–123; for premenstrual syndrome (PMS), 101

hearing loss, ear infections and, 84

heartburn, ginger for treating, 39

heart conditions/diseases: cautions about, 35, 56; treatments for, 29, 41, 44

Heart of Herbs (school), 3

heavy periods, 101–102; treatments for: herbal remedies, 101–102; *Profuse Menstruation Regulation Blend,* 166–167; specific herbs: American cranesbill, 101; beth root, 101; cinnamon, 101; lady's mantle, 101; periwinkle, 101; red raspberry leaf, 101; shepherd's purse, 101; yarrow, 101; yellow dock root, 101

helichrysum *(Helichrysum angustifolia),* 40–41, 98

Helichrysum angustifolia (helichrysum), 40–41, 98

hemlock, 10, 61

hemorrhage, herb for treating, 28

hemorrhoids, treatments for: American cranesbill, 28; chickweed, 33; cypress, 36; greater celandine, 40; mullein, 45; passionflower, 47; white oak bark, 56; witch hazel leaf, 57

herbal baths: essential oils for, 121, 123; specific herbs for: burdock, 86–87; calendula, 71; chamomile, 71; chickweed, 33; ginger, 70, 88; lavender, 70, 71, 93; marshmallow, 86–87; oats, 46, 70; oregano, 71; red clover, 85; rosemary, 71; rosewood, 51; slippery elm, 70; tea tree, 51; yarrow, 86–87; yellow dock, 86–87

Herbal Cough Syrup, 72

herbalism, 7–8. *See also* safety of herbs; author's, 1, 2;

for children, 3–5, 8–9; history of, 9; learning about, 12, 15; styles of, 19–22; timeline of, 10–11

herbalists: essential oils prescribed by, 121; finding, 17–18; for flu remedy consultations, 89; historical, 10–11; learning from, 15; names of, 2–3; questions to ask of, 18–19

Herbal Therapy and Supplements: A Scientific and Traditional Approach (Kuhn and Winston), 12

herb gardens, 181–186; purpose patches, 185–186; sacred garden, 181–183; seasonal gardens, 183–184

herb gatherer's saying, 107

herpes/herpes simplex/herpes zoster, treatments for: black walnut, 30; burdock, 31; elder, 37; licorice, 43; oats, 46; thuja, 55

hibiscus *(Hibiscus sabdariffa),* 41

Hibiscus sabdariffa (hibiscus), 41

high blood pressure, 29, 43, 51

HIV, elder and, 37

hives, oats for treating, 46

Hobbs, Christopher, 2

Hoffmann, David, 2; *Holistic Herbal,* 12

Holistic Herbal (Hoffmann), 12

Homemade Ginger Tea, 83, 156

homeopathy/homeopathic treatments, 17, 21; for colic, 75; for conjunctivitis, 77; for teething, 95

honey, caution about, for babies, 142

Honey, Garlic, 73, 169

hops *(Humulus lupulus),* 41, 59, 182

horehound *(Marrubium vulgare),* 41–42

hormonal imbalances: dysmenorrhea (painful period) and, 99; heavy periods and, 101; treatments for, 50, 57

horseradish *(Armoracia rusticana),* 42; cautions about, 126, 187; nutrition and, 187; for sinus congestion, 73

horsetail *(Equisetum arvense),* 65, 94, 182

Humulus lupulus (hops), 41, 59, 182

Hydrastis canadensis (goldenseal). *See* goldenseal *(Hydrastis canadensis)*

hygiene, 71, 95

hyperactivity, skullcap for treating, 51

Hypericum perforatum (St. John's wort). *See* St. John's wort *(Hypericum perforatum)*

hypoglycemia, geranium essential oil and, caution about, 122

hypotensives, 26, 39

hyptertension, licorice and, caution about, 43

hyssop *(Hyssopus officinalis),* 44; cautions about, 121, 122; in garden, 182

Hyssop officinalis (hyssop). *See* hyssop *(Hyssopus officinalis)*

I

identifying herbs, 23

immune system: astragalus and, caution about, 29; colds and, 71; disease/illness and, 63, 71; thrush and, 95; treatments for: antimicrobials, 26; herbal remedies: *Immunity Tonic Tea,* 89, 139; *Immunity Tonic Tincture,* 140; specific herbs: astragalus, 29; boneset, 31; burdock, 31; echinacea, 36, 84;

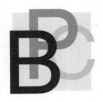

BOOK PUBLISHING COMPANY

since 1974—books that educate, inspire, and empower

To find sprouting seeds and other vegan favorites online, visit:
www.healthy-eating.com

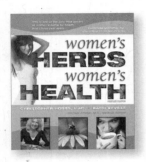

Women's Herbs, Women's Health
Christopher Hobbs, LAc,
Kathi Keville
978-1-57067-152-4
$24.95

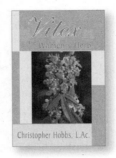

Vitex, The Women's Herb
Christopher Hobbs, LAc,
978-1-57067-157-9
$7.95

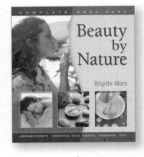

Beauty by Nature
Complete Body Care
Brigitte Mars
978-1-57067-193-7
$19.95

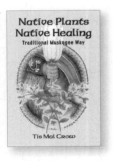

Native Plants, Native Healing
Tis Mal Crow
978-1-57067-105-0
$12.95

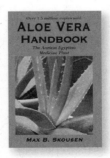

Aloe Vera Handbook
Max B. Skousen
978-1-57067-196-2
$3.95

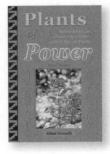

Plants of Power
Alfred Savinelli
978-1-57067-130-2
$11.95